MW00423382

Sensual Healing

Sensual Healing

AN ELEMENTAL GUIDE
TO FEELING GOOD

TERESA KENNEDY

M. EVANS AND COMPANY, INC.
New York

Copyright © 1996 by Teresa Kennedy

All rights reserved. No part of this book may be reproduced
or transmitted in any form or by any means without the
written permission of the publisher.

M. Evans and Company, Inc.
216 East 49th Street
New York, New York 10017

ISBN: 0-87131-806-7

Designed and type formatting by Bernard Schleifer

Manufactured in the United States of America

For my dear friend and editor
Betty Anne Crawford
Feel better!
and
For my mother
Virginia Weber Kennedy
a master of healing
who taught me the
power of joy.

Contents

Introduction

IT IS POSSIBLE TO ENSURE YOUR PHYSICAL AND EMOTIONAL well-being, increase your attractiveness, involvement, and, yes, even your spiritual awareness through the systemic regular, moderated indulgence of your five senses. The healing system presented in this book is completely different from the usual strict regimen of self-denial, will power, and low-grade suffering offered by most holistic healing programs.

The art and practice of healing as expressed in this work depends upon the integration and reintegration of the spiritual, physical, and emotional aspects of life as expressed through elemental energy. It is a system that is both very old and very new, utilizing the five senses—touch, taste, sight, sound, and smell—as keys to both the inner and outer worlds.

The word healing comes from the old English word for whole. Wellness, then, can be thought of as wholeness. And wholeness is easier to set as a goal and to achieve as a reality if we accept the sensuality of our true natures, and accept ourselves as beings sensorily and sensually equipped to dwell within a cosmos where physical reality can and does have a spiritual life. In fact, the ability to tap into the spiritual energy of the physical world and to align oneself with that energy is what wholeness is all about.

The demands of life in the modern world have caused many of us to shut our senses down, decrease our awareness, and lessen our natural sensitivity as we struggle to avoid stress, pressure, and the illness they can cause. Yet, in doing so, we also turn ourselves off from the worlds of simple pleasure—available to us through heightened sensory awareness—and deny ourselves access to real vitality. We lose touch with our true natures, becoming alienated from others, lacking or disordered in our personal energy fields, and, finally, ill.

Yet, it has been scientifically proven that simple laughter increases the endorphin levels in the bloodstream, speeds up cell regeneration, and dissolves even cancerous tumors; that the so-called "placebo effect" can have a significant bearing on your health and well-being; and that, ultimately, attitiudes of mind have real and measurable effects on the condition of the body.

Thus it can be said that by indulging in pleasurable feelings and sensations you can prevent, treat, and heal illness. If you feel good, you look better, live longer, and are capable of increased general productivity. Consider that the more relaxed Type B personality is less likely to fall victim to heart disease than the more driven Type A. Or that the simple practice of meditation and conscious relaxation can alleviate back pain and head aches, and reduce high blood pressure and the risk of stroke and heart disease.

This book will help you determine which of the four elements—Earth, Fire, Air, and Water—is your dominant type and, based on your elemental profile, offers the best therapy for your personality including recommendations for color therapy, aromatherapy, crystal therapy, and sound therapy, as well as massage, diet, and relaxation techniques. Meditations and affirmations for each element personality are included, along with fine-tuned variations for elemental rulership combinations. By surrounding yourself with healing and energizing objects, sights, scents, tastes, and sounds, you can make full use of sensory input to facilitate mental, physical, emotional, and spiritual healing. Each elemental section also includes a monthly tune-up sensory healing program designed to cleanse, strengthen, and renew.

By bringing a wide range of healing arts and therapies together and grouping them according to elemental energy and rulership, I hope to give readers ways to nourish and heal their bioelectric fields—to align themselves with the rhythms of life on this planet and to encourage the notion that self-indulgence in the form of physical and sensory pleasure should be thought of as a necessary and valid nourishment on the soul's journey to wellness, wholeness, and spiritual awareness.

Finally, I want to encourage the idea that healing through the senses should be part and parcel of the way you live your life, not just something to be hauled out when you are ill, emotionally exhausted, or spiritually spent. The sensory pleasures and elemental nourishments suggested in these pages are aesthetically pleasing, non-invasive, and readily available for little money. They are offered in the hope that they will be used and incorporated into your life because they make you feel good, give you pleasure, and are invaluable in the prevention of a breakdown in your energy field in the form of physical or emotional illness. By making these routines part of your daily life, these methods will increase your personal power, your awareness of yourself and others, and will allow you to receive the blessings of a benevolent universe.

Sensual Healing

Sexual Healing

The Core of Being

MOST READERS ARE ALREADY AWARE THAT IN WESTERN astrological tradition the twelve signs of the zodiac are ruled by the four elements of earth, air, fire, and water. Eastern astrological tradition also works on a system of elements, but does not use the element of air, adding instead the elements of metal and wood. For purposes of this volume, however, we will be concerned with determining the elemental rulers of the individual chart under the Western system only.

For those unfamiliar with the elemental rulers of the twelve signs, they are:

FIRE: Aries, Leo, and Sagittarius
EARTH: Taurus, Virgo, and Capricorn
WATER: Cancer, Scorpio, and Pisces
AIR: Gemini, Libra, and Aquarius

Elements have also been traditionally associated with the planets themselves:

FIRE: Sun, Mars
EARTH: Saturn, Pluto
WATER: Moon, Venus, and Neptune
AIR: Mercury, Uranus

The concept of the elements governing personality types and areas of human endeavor is not new, and can be found throughout a long history of ancient mystical and modern psychological theory. In the Tarot, for example, the four elements are seen to correspond to the four suits of the Lower Arcana—wands to fire, pentacles to earth, cups to water, and swords to air. The elements were also thought to rule the four medieval humors, or types of personality: choleric being ruled by fire, phelgmatic ruled by earth, sanguine ruled by air, and melancholic ruled by water.

As more modern systems of thought emerge, the idea of elemental rulership holds sway. Under the Jungian system of psychology, there exist four basic types—intuitive, sensation-oriented, thinking, and feeling, still corresponding to the elements of fire, earth, air, and water respectively.

So an element can be thought of as nothing more or less than a particular kind of energy. The four elements are the basic foundation for the material and organic world—the laws by which our universe can be said to operate. They are, in effect, the language of energy. And though each of us can be said to be dominated by a particular kind of energy or element, each of us necessarily requires the influence of the other three.

Why utilize so ancient a system in the modern world? Because, from an evolutionary point of view, we *are* ancient man in many significant ways. One has only to study the rise in such disorders as chemical depression, Attention Deficit Disorder, ulcers, and stress-related disease to understand that while technology, science, and medicine have evolved far beyond the wildest imaginings of even a hundred years ago, the human organism has yet to evolve to the point at which it can develop the coping mechanisms to deal with the pressures of life in a technological universe. Our brain chemistry, our physical bodies, and our psychological makeup have not changed very much in tens of thousands of years. It behooves us, then, to study the ancient ways for the knowledge and understanding these very old systems can bring to our lives. If the ancients understood the value of keeping one's personal energy properly aligned with universal rhythms and currents, perhaps we can take that same knowledge and apply it to ourselves with great benefit. As organisms, we remain what might be called artifacts of an earlier time. We can therefore benefit from the same disciplines, practices, and theories that helped our ancient ancestors.

And while many Western astrologers neglect or overlook the importance of the four elemental energies as not being in keeping with a "scientific" perspective, or as simply being too obvious to talk about, most healing systems do not. Indian Ayurvedic medicine, Hatha Yoga, Chinese acupuncture and herbalism and its modern cousin, aromatherapy, all address the issue of element as central to health and wholeness.

Why is your elemental ruler so important? Because it is your identifying energy. The ruling element of the individual chart can tell us where that person's life force truly resides, and how it is expressed through the course of his or her lifetime. Your ruling element can be thought of as your personal energy field. It can show you how you are attuned to the universal energy. And, by employing and practicing the healing methods most compatible with your element, you are in effect feeding your energy field in the most positive possible way—amplifying your basic life force to the degree that you will be better able to resist disease, stress, and psychological and physical disorders. That is healing at the most basic—and sometimes most effective—level.

Finding Your Ruling Element

For most people, it is easy to establish the nature of your ruling energy: All you need to know is the ruling elment of your sun sign. Aries, Leo, and Sagittarius are the Fire signs; Taurus, Virgo, and Capricorn are the Earth signs; Cancer, Scorpio, and Pisces are the Water signs; and Gemini, Libra, and Aquarius are the Air signs. If you want to find out if you have a combination or qualifying energy, it helps to know your rising and moon signs as well. Obviously, someone born under the sign of Leo, with the moon in Aries and Sagittarius rising, is ruled predominantly by the element of Fire. But how about someone with the sun in Libra, Pisces rising, and a Cancer moon? The rising sign and the moon signs are both in Water, even though the sun is in Air. So we would call this person an Air/Water personality. A person with the sun in the neighboring sign of Scorpio, Pisces rising, and a Libra moon, on the other hand, would probably be considered a Water/Air personality. But given the fact that this person has a heavy water influence, we could discern that the Air element of the personality needed regular healing and augmentation, so that the more intellectual aspects of this personality are not consistently overwhelmed by their more emotional qualities.

But if, after determining your elemental ruler, you don't feel your profile fits even with qualifying energies, you may want to refer to the information provided in the Astrological Keys section, beginning on page 189, for some deeper interpretive analysis.

Finally, always let your intuition play a significant role in determining your own or someone else's elemental profile. Keep in mind that these elements came to be associated with personality and destiny because they were seen, over and over again, to correspond with certain qualities of the soul.

Healing and Balance

Most mystical, holistic, and alternative healing traditions address the concept of balance. Under many of these systems, healing (and thereby wholeness) is thought to be achieved by augmenting certain energies, or using healing methods to add an element in some material form to the environment or energy field of someone lacking that element. By giving the individual access and exposure to tools and therapies believed to be associated with the element or quality of energy they seem to lack, it is thought that blocked energy is released, absent energy is supplied, and thus the possibility of disease and any chronic emotional and physical problems can be reduced or even eliminated.

But it is my own belief, based on observation, that before any healer begins to address the issue of balance, it is equally important to find the right approach—to adjust the proposed healing therapy to the character and temperament of the individual. The goal of spiritual healing should be to identify and center the Self—to realign and reconcile an individual's spiritual, mental, and physical energies in such a way that the Self (in the highest sense) is able to quite literally *be* itself, unhampered by blockages, fears, emotional baggage, and even physical discomfort.

No one, for example, is ever going to successfully balance a fiery temperament by pouring water on it, in either a literal or figurative sense. Better to accept and to encourage the Fire personality to learn to acknowledge that the roller coaster ride of their emotional life is part and parcel of who they are and why they are here. No method of healing contained in this book is given with an eye to working miracles. What these methods can do for our fiery individual is to help him or her appreciate the nature of the ride; to stay centered within his or her frequent emotional storms; and not to be overwhelmed by their own—or others'— passions.

If the goal of healing, then, is to be getting and keeping in touch with the soul—the inner life force that dwells within each of us—it only makes sense to confine oneself to therapies and exercises that make the outer self comfortable, happy, and clear from unwanted outside influences. Therapies and exercises that at the outset are not in harmony with a person's nature, temperament, and inclinations are not going to do very much for that person. Thus, an overemphasis on "balance" can be counterproductive if we do not consider the true nature of the individual involved.

Healing and the Senses

It is the central premise of this book that the five senses—sight, hearing, taste, touch, and smell can be access points to both the inner and outer worlds. Consider your own personality: Are you visual? Verbal? Do you respond to the things of the earth or are you more excited and stimulated by the world of ideas and concepts? Are you sensual? Ascetic? Esoteric? Which gives you more pleasure, the color blue or the scent of peppermint? Is your favorite way to relax to curl up against a fuzzy sheepskin or to run around the block and work up a sweat?

Obviously, the answers to these questions and others like it will not all be the same, nor will they be the same for one person all the time. Yet, it is the senses that can give us real cues to the true nature of not just our physical, but also our spiritual needs.

To truly keep in touch with the sensual experiences that give you genuine pleasure is perhaps the first step on the road to true healing, wholeness, and wellness. Someone who really feels good, looks good, is happier, more functional, healthier, and, finally, more spiritually aware than the person who has lost track of the function of something as simple as the regular activation of their own pleasure centers.

"No pain, no gain" is the popular wisdom for attaining wellness, and one that has its roots in the idea that denial of the flesh is the only way to spiritual enlightenment. But one has only to open a newspaper or watch the nightly news to realize that the denial of pleasure is indeed a finite system. The list of all the things we are supposed to deny ourselves in the interest of good health grows daily, and much of the evidence to support these theories is entirely contradictory.

While there is certainly a case to be made for moderation, human beings are simply not geared for constant denial. To attempt to deny the body food, sleep, leisure, and so forth results in elevated stress levels, depression, and finally physical manifestations of spiritual "disease." In addition, modern life provides a kind of regular, nonpleasureable assault upon the senses. Environmental factors, such as noise, pollution, overcrowding, and urban blight, along with a general overemphasis on function and an underemphasis on aesthetics, all contribute to the shutting down of our senses—and the closing off of our access points to the inner self as we seek to protect it from such assault.

Denied the nourishment of pleasure, the being, the soul within the body, becomes shut off from the body—

uncomfortable with itself to the point where physical dysfunction is all but inevitable.

When taken to an elemental level in spiritual healing, this means only that certain personality types are more sensually responsive to certain tools, exercises, and therapies than others. The elemental route is but a highly useful shortcut to the activation of pleasure centers through the senses.

A slow-moving Earth type, for example, is not "healed" nor necessarily balanced by fiery risk-taking— only further stressed. Nor does it make sense to instruct an Air-dominated personality to undertake long sessions of meditation or progressive relaxation exercises. Though they may indeed need to relax, Air types are simply too mentally restless to "stop thinking" or "make your mind a blank" on command.

In using elements in healing, then, it is critical to know how each of the elements are associated with specific areas of soul and being. Below is a short summary for each element's domain and personality type. More detailed descriptions of each type and combination types are found in subsequent chapters.

Fire: Rules the passions. Energy, enthusiasm, ardor, and an essential optimism can all be said to characterize the Fire personality. The true Fire personality seems able to activate others through sheer force of will. Relentless and active, Fire never says die, and they can cherish a secret belief in their own invincibility. Usually honest, always straightforward, Fire personalities can display an almost naive quality when dealing with the world at large. Self-centered and even quite gaudily selfish at times, they are nonetheless perennially optimistic, traveling through life at breakneck speed.

Yet Fire needs fuel. These personalities are forever in search of the new. They are considered pioneers because fire illuminates; they are considered jealous and possessive because fire consumes. They are generous and open-hearted because at its best, fire warms and protects. The key to healing the Fire personality is only to remember that it is often difficult to tell one passion from another when one stands at the center of the flame. Independent to a fault, Fire is both the least able to introspect, and the least able to consider others able to help with their problems.

Earth: Rules the senses. That which can be felt, seen, touched, tasted, and smelled all fall under the auspices of earth. These are the most "realistic" of personalities, quite literally "grounded" in material and sensual reality. Earth people are the builders, the acquirers, the owners—the most perennially stable of all the element types. Earth shelters, earth is naturally organized, and earth changes only by slow degrees. They can be considered the most at home of any of the personality types, quite comfortable in their bodies, and usually nearly impervious to stress. But Earth rarely takes chances. Slow-moving by nature, it is easy for them to get mired as slow movement slows down to no movement at all. Cautious, dignified and even calculating, Earth seeks permanence in relationships and environment. In healing Earth, remember only "Earth to earth, ashes to ashes, dust to dust," thereby reminding the Earth-ruled that even the biggest empire, the grandest bank account, and the most stable of relationships are, at best, transitory in the light of eternity.

Air: Rules the mind, the intellect, the world of ideas. Thought processes, language, and communication are the hallmarks of the Air personality. Concepts are more important to Air than the details of life and as such they can sometimes be considered to be long on inspiration but decidedly short on the perspiration part of bringing their ideas into more concrete forms of reality. Air is restless and changeable, difficult to contain or pin down. Air's intellect and natural sophistication can sometimes seem dispassionate or even cold to more emotionally sensitive types, resulting in Air's sense of isolation from others. Yet Air people can no more keep themselves from analyzing life than the wind can itself keep from blowing—they live to communicate. Air types are frequently susceptible to insomnia, nervous disorders, and stress-related illness, all resulting from mental overload. Air has gained a somewhat unfair reputation for being shallow; far from it. Air is simply faster than other people. People can be met, absorbed, thought through, enjoyed, digested, and discarded in the time it takes a cautious Earth type to decide to give out his or her phone number or a Water-ruled personality to identify his or her feelings. Remember: In any situation, Air is in it for what they can learn and subsequently communicate to others, just as seeds are picked up by the wind, carried to another place and planted. They can be obsessive about solving all the little puzzles of life, going over the details again and again. In healing Air, consider that without variety and circulation, air can become stale, stagnant, and unbreathable in very short order.

Water: Rules the emotions, the world of feeling. Sensitivity is its hallmark, and Water personalities tend to communicate best in nonverbal ways. These souls are affected by life's smallest incidents in the same way water is disturbed by a skipping stone. Perhaps it is because of this quality that Water types dislike a linear world. They excel in the arts and creative endeavors of all kinds and flourish in nonstructured environments. Yet, these impressionable souls tend to seek structure and stability, often to their own detriment. Wonderfully sympathetic, there is no better type to turn to when the chips are down, yet it is equally easy for a Water type to have such a degree of empathy and sympathy for his fellows that he or she becomes quite weighed down by the problems of others. Water tends to absorb the identities of others without ever becoming quite sure of its own, and as a result can gain a reputation for being deceptive and unreliable. Not so. Water merely understands, better than any other type, that reality—like emotion—is flexible, changing according to point of view, environment, and the currents of unseen feeling that are its domain. For that reason, they are by far the most adept of the personality types at rediscovering and reinventing their lives, simply by changing their points of view. Water types can be highly opinionated, however, and quite impervious to "logical" arguments once they have made up their minds. In healing Water, remember that it is water's nature to move on—they must be freed from a tendency to cling to worn-out life situations, relationships, and jobs simply because they feel they are needed or somehow dependent upon a particular circumstance for stability. Fresh water nourishes all things. Stagnant water is no good to anyone.

The Elemental Relationships

The elements are further classified according to "masculine" and "feminine" energies—the active and the passive; the creative and receptive; the yin and yang qualities of their specific energies. Fire and Air are considered "masculine," while Earth and Water are considered "feminine" types of energy. From a purely psychological point of view, Fire and Air energy can be thought of as self-expressive, while Earth and Water can be thought of as self-repressive.

In determining an individual's elemental profile, however, it is perhaps more important to be concerned with the relationships the elements have to one another. Some elements are naturally complimentary, some not so. At its simplest air feeds fire; water nourishes earth. But what of the relationship between air and water? Air can evaporate water, but having done so, will water not return as rain? Earth can smother fire, but does it not also warm it? Just as relationships in nature contain potential for creation and destruction, so do the elemental relationships of the individual chart. Those with natural contradictions within their core personality profiles should view such tendencies not as self-defeating, but, properly reconciled, as creative opportunities for healing and wholeness.

The Absence of an Element (or Elements)

The complete absence of an element or elements in a chart will also have a bearing on an individual's response to healing. While it is not, as previously mentioned, necessary to begin by attempting to "balance" the lack of a certain kind of energy, noting the weakness or absence of a particular type of energy in a chart can do much to illuminate and complete the elemental profile of an individual and help to illuminate the best approach to their healing needs.

Fire Weakness

The primary characteristic of Fire weakness in a chart can be seen in the fact that these individuals need more rest than other people. They tend to shyness and to be rather generally retiring, preferring to remain on the sidelines, rather than at center stage. Healing exercises that encourage the creation of a peaceful interlude spent in solitude at some point during the day or night are especially beneficial. Fire-weak types are observers by nature, but they can be quite easily worn out and down by the subtle, invisible influences of other personalities, the environment, and their own daily routines. They tend to lack a sense of *joie de vivre*, and Fire weakness will almost always indicate a tendency to hang on to problems, injuries, and hurts. They are literally slower to heal than any other group.

Earth Weakness

Earth-weak personalities are characterized by a certain naiveté when it comes to the affairs of day-to-day living. They have a "lost in space" quality that can appear to others as utter and even deliberate irresponsibility. But in truth, it is simply difficult for these personalities to track the myriad details of keeping the bills paid, the floors swept, and the clocks wound. Healing therapies that involve a particular object or routine can be quite useful, since it will help the person to focus their sometimes quite scattered energies. They are apt to ignore the needs of the physical form, and can fall ill due to simple neglect. These are the people who forget to sleep, to exercise, or to eat.

Water Weakness

The Water-weak personality can seem a curious case due to the fact that they are quite genuinely less emotional than other people, to the point of being downright callous or cold. They almost always can be found to have a certain sardonic sense of humor, however, and can be looked to for both old-fashioned "horse sense" and superior observational and organizational skills. Healing methods that are well-organized, focused, and highly evolved conceptually will be of most merit. From the purely physical standpoint, those with too little Water will almost always suffer from the tendency to accumulate toxicity in the body. Water cleanses and purges. And so Water-weak people need, more than any other type, to drink those eight to ten glasses of water per day.

Air Weakness

While an Air-weak individual will almost always be dependent upon others for mental stimulation, it is best to keep in mind that these individuals are slow to communicate in verbal ways. Thus, healing exercises that involve complicated concepts, directions, or verbal communications will be less than useful. A series of chants, for example, will be of little use to the Air-weak type, since verbal expression is more of a chore than a pleasure. They take the world quite personally most times and can tend to the sentimental (this type probably carried around a security blanket as a child), so it is best to focus healing methods around personal favorites—colors, pieces of familiar music, and the like. Air-weak people are subject to nervous exhaustion, due to an excessive tendency to worry. They are out of touch with their bodies, yet tend to react to a threatening new concept or idea by physically manifesting their rebellion in some kind of illness. Migraines and allergies particularly afflict this group.

The Senses and the House Quadrants

The methods, practices, and various disciplines of alternative healing methods can be overwhelming. Color healing, music healing, chants, visualization, crystal and gemstone therapies, herbs, candle burning, and the like can seem terribly confusing to the uninitiated. Yet it is important to keep in mind that most healing disciplines all have essentially the same objective— to more properly align the inner and outer beings, to establish regular communication between the soul and the body, and to more fully integrate the myriad aspects of life into a functional healthy and happy whole. The trick, if indeed there is a trick, is to hit upon that method that works for you. And while many readers have and will continue to experience false starts in trying and discarding the exercises and methods described in these pages, rest assured that there is something that will, with time and practice, work for you.

But to enable you to find the right method a little faster, you might do well to consider a final factor in determining the best approach to healing through the individual elemental profile—by charting the most responsive sense or senses according to the position of planets and elemental domination in a specific area of the natal chart. Since there are, of course, five senses and only four quadrants in the circle of the zodiac, it is not a perfect system, but it can quite adequately serve as a kind of compass to the most highly developed of the senses in an individual profile.

Specifically, highly visual people can be found when there is a preponderance of planets (particularly the sun) in the ninth, tenth, or eleventh houses. Here you will find visual artists, architects, and designers of all kinds. Taken a step further, those with most of their planets in the northern, or upper half, of the chart will generally respond better to visually-oriented therapies than those who have no planets there.

Continuing around the circle, those with a preponderance of planets in what might be called the northeast portion of the chart are also visual yet will almost always display a more highly developed sense of color, which graduates to a highly developed tactile sense at the easternmost point of the chart, the twelfth to first house cusp. Here, then, is where approaches like crystal therapy might be considered, since crystals are both colorful and tactile.

Pure eastern people generally can be considered to have a more highly developed tactile sense than their western counterparts and do well with therapies that involve objects or talismans they can touch, hold, and use to focus their energies, or to those therapies that involve prolonged tactile sensation, such as massage.

Southeast people continue to respond to touch but begin to be influenced by the sense of smell. Prominent planets here would indicate adding scented oils to the massage perhaps, or burning incense. Perfumes and aromatherapy work well in general for people with planets in the southern half of the chart, culminating at the third to fourth house cusp. Naturally, a Water person with southern planets would benefit from healing baths employing aromatherapy oils, while an Earth personality might want to skip the bath, but sit down to his or her session of meditation enveloped in the scent of a nearby bouquet of flowers or eucalyptus.

As we begin to move north again and into the western half of the chart we find the rulership of taste and sound. Southwest people, that is, those with planets in a latter portion of the fourth, the fifth, and early degrees of the sixth will all be food and drink lovers—the presence of earth here will augment the tendency. Thus herbal infusions, teas, elixirs, and salads of fresh herbs will be particularly effective in healing. Those with a heavy planetary presence in the late sixth, seventh, and eighth house will generally display a more highly developed auditory sense than their eastern counterparts and will respond to music, chants, and sound more readily than some others. The lower the western placement, the more personal the musical selections should be. Northwest people, on the other hand, might consider music with a more technical, even mathematical construction; the works of J. S. Bach, for example, might be a good choice while at the same time beginning to incorporate some visual elements.

Obviously, there are no hard and fast rules for considering planetary and elemental house placement in relation to the five senses, but a glance at the most heavily populated signs and houses can be a good indicator of just which of the five senses to begin with when determining appropriate individual healing methods.

The Means and Methods of Sensual Healing

THIS REFERENCE SECTION IS INCLUDED TO FAMILIARIZE the reader with some of the most commonly used techniques, objects, and practices used in alternative and spiritual healing. Each category includes a brief description, history, common uses, and the spiritual and physical functions of the discipline.

This list is by no means comprehensive; it is meant only to be an introduction to the wealth of myth, literature, and folklore that comprise the rich and varied traditions of alternative healing practice. Recipes, methods, and directions have been included where appropriate, but do remember that by far the most vital ingredient for the success of any such therapy or formula is the investment and concentration of your own energy and power in its success.

Nothing included in these pages will hurt you—barring the odd allergic reaction—and most of these formulas will help you. But it is a salient characteristic of most of these traditions that they tend to work better and faster when the practitioner believes that they are going to work. Most alternative healing therapies focus on the concept of wholeness. The healthy and happy individual is considered to be more "whole" than his or her stressed out, unhappy, or unwell counterpart. If the aspects of the self—mind, body, and spirit—are aligned and in tune with one another, wellness results. Thus, the practice of such therapies should include the faith and willingness to believe in the value of wholeness as an attainable goal.

Nor is anything here meant to be considered a substitute for modern medicine. Unlike many who have written on such subjects, I do not propose that traditional Western medicine and alternative healing practice are mutually exclusive.

But even as Western medicine has begun to acknowledge the effect of the mind, spirit, and emotions on the physical form, I do propose to anyone interested in trying any of the remedies included here that their effectiveness is sure to be considerably enhanced if you happen to believe in what you're doing. Just as an antibiotic series won't prove particularly effective if you don't take the prescribed amount, don't take it every day, or simply don't have any faith in an antibiotic's ability to cure what ails you, a daily dose of chamomile infusion isn't going to do a thing for your insomnia if you don't allow it to help you.

And while no one is asking that you put your faith in anything you haven't tried and found to be effective, an attitude of concentration, willingness, and openness, along with a measure of healthy curiosity in experimenting with these formulas is certainly welcome and appropriate. The efficacy of any healing potion, infusion, or practice is necessarily going to be severely limited when the individual's own power to heal himself or others is blocked by skepticism, carelessness, or something as simple as a failure to follow directions for preparation or dosage. Thus, the addition of a measure of the practitioner's own personal power in the preparation and practice of any of these healing solutions is a welcome and necessary ingredient for its success.

Aromatherapy

While the term aromatherapy was first coined in France in the early twentieth century by physician R. M. Gattefosse, the use of plants and plant essences is as old as mankind. Early cave paintings show the inclusion of flowers at burial sites and tell of the use of plants in medicine.

The practice of aromatherapy, or the use of fragrant essences to affect mood and health, probably has it roots in ancient Egypt, though some texts point to its probable use in the lost civilizations of Atlantis and Lemuria. The Egyptians, however, have documented the use of balsamic substances, scented barks and resins, oils, and perfumes in medicine and embalming.

The Greeks were the first westerners to transform the practice of healing into more of a science than a superstition. Nevertheless, a central premise of Hippocrates' regime for good health made use of a daily scented bath and aromatic massage, both of which are central to today's aromatherapeutic practice.

The use of aromatics and essential oils to ward off disease and improve health continued to be practiced throughout the Middle Ages and well into the late eighteenth century. Most households cultivated their own herb or "paradise" gardens, as they were called, rather than relying on finding herbs in the wild. But as chemistry began to come into its own, chemical and synthetic medicines began to take the place of natural remedies. As a result, aromatherapy, along with its cousin herbalism, or phytotherapy, was displaced until the relatively recent resurgence of interest in the subject.

Specifically, aromatherapy contends that scent affects mood, mind, and body, both through its employment in the environment—in such things as incense, air fresheners, scented baths, and perfumes— and through its application in what the French call "soft" medicine—the ingestion of scented teas or infusions, the application of essential oils that are absorbed through the skin, and so forth—to remedy specific ailments and complaints. However, it should be remembered that much of what is marketed today under the auspices of "aromatherapy" is a far cry from the intended uses and medicinal factors purported to be associated with natural plants and essences.

Quality control is truly important in aromatherapy. Synthetic essences or essences that have been corrupted, either by the addition of other scents and fillers or by chemical fertilizers and pesticides, naturally affect the remedial properties of the product. Since substances like essential oils are not labeled as to their ingredients or chemical composition, it is doubly important to check with your dealer as to the authenticity and purity of any product, or better still, to make your own if you have access to organically grown herbs and flowers. If you prefer to buy, look to two single factors when purchasing essential oils: (1) Essential oils lose their volatility quite easily, and should always be stored in dark brown bottles. Don't buy any bottle that isn't dark brown or that looks dusty or old. (2) Essential oils are really quite expensive, especially when dealing with a well-known, reputable dealer or perfumer. Be prepared to pay handsomely, secure in the knowledge that one does indeed get what one pays for, i.e., the genuine essence, not a laboratory synthesized imitation.

Modern perfumers divide fragrance into one of three categories. The pure or "virginal" scents derived from citrons, lavender, and mints are found in such things as soap, household cleaning products, and the like. "Masculine" fragrances are warmer and spicier, including clove, pine, civet, and patchouli. Lastly the so-called "feminine" fragrances are more exotic and sensual and are derived from rose, ambergris, musk, and jasmine. Yet these three classifications are in fact derived from the older astrological system of scent classification. As the planets were thought to exert positive and negative influence on our daily lives, so it was thought to be beneficial to surround yourself and your environs with such fragrances as could "draw" the energies of a particular planet.

Saturn rules cypress and myrrh
Jupiter rules nutmeg, clove, cinnamon, and saffron
Mars rules pine, camphor, and pepperwort
Venus rules rose, myrtle, and violet
The Sun rules bay, frankincense, and rosemary
The Moon rules lilies and jasmine
Mercury rules lavender, marjoram, and cinnamon

Naturally, it was thought most beneficial to surround onself with fragrances that spoke to the influences of the "happier" planets like the sun, Mercury, Jupiter, and Venus. Whether or not you believe that herbs and essences can draw specific planetary influences, the idea that fragrances have beneficial effects upon both the psychology and physiology of human beings is one that may go in and out of fashion, but has never entirely gone away.

From a purely elemental perspective, the use of fragrance both in aromatherapy and in natural plant form is a wonderful way of attuning and nourishing your personal energies. Do experiment and mix elementally attuned scents to achieve a truly personal perfume for yourself or a friend, and remember that, like crystals, you may find yourself responding to a particular scent while in a particular state of mind, then moving on to another. Initially however, it is best to choose your essences, fragrances, and scents to correspond with your elemental ruler by referring to the chart on the facing page.

Scents of the Elements

EARTH SCENTS

Cedar, cypress, sandalwood, apple, woodruff, oakmoss, cinnamon, vanilla, nutmeg, patchouli, vetivert, carnation, lilac, mimosa, myrrh, and thyme.

AIR SCENTS

Mints, lily of the valley, lemongrass, licorice, marjoram, myrtle, dill, parsley, sweet pea, verbena, peony, iris, chamomile, geranium, lemon verbena, and anise.

FIRE SCENTS

Saffron, bay, lemon balm, frankincense, ginger, lime, nasturtium, calendula, basil, neroli, pennyroyal, marigold, angelica, heliotrope, and rosemary.

WATER SCENTS

Freesia, gardenia, jasmine, hyacinth, narcissus, rose, lily, mugwort, ylang-ylang, daisy, gooseberry, tansy, violet, cherry, and poppy.

To Make Herb or Fragrance Oil:

Homemade herb oil will naturally not be as strong as a commercially distilled product, but will nonetheless prove effective in most of the therapies suggested in later chapters, and will never threaten your health in the manner that some synthetic or commercially blended oils can.

Harvest, wash, and dry the fresh herbs. Dried herbs can also be used, but will yield a product of less strength and essence than one made with fresh herbs. Use 8 ounces of fresh herbs or 4 ounces of dried herbs to 2 cups of grapeseed or soy oil, both of which are readily available in health-food stores. Shred or bruise the herb lightly and place in a clear glass container. Cover with the oil, cover the container, and place on a sunny windowsill for three weeks, turning and shaking the bottle from time to time. Strain the oil and decant into dark bottles. Store in the refrigerator if possible, though the scent of some oils can affect other foods. Otherwise, a cool dark cupboard or root cellar will suffice. Dispose of any unused oils after six months.

Bath Therapies

The use of the bath as a healing therapy probably dates from the Egyptians as well, and has come down to us through history in forms as simple as that of a handful of rosebuds in the water, to the alternating hot and cold of steam baths and saunas, to technology-assisted baths like the jacuzzi.

The appeal of the bath is multifaceted; there is the sensual appeal of the skin in contact with the water, the cleansing and detoxifying properties, and the added attraction of removing oneself from other activities simply to enjoy time alone for a good, long soak or steam. Additionally, baths can be engineered to meet individual needs with the addition of oils, bubbles, or salts to enhance a bath's relaxing, cleansing, or invigorating qualities. Specific essential oils can be absorbed through the skin in a bath to meet special medicinal or emotional needs as well. Healing baths that are specific to the elemental types are included in later chapters, but the following is a good, all-purpose "recipe" for all-over aura and body cleansing and detoxification.

Balancing Energy Bath

Under open taps, toss ½ cup sea salt, ½ cup baking soda, 6 drops of violet oil, 1 cinnamon stick, and a handful of fresh sage leaves. Soak at least 20 minutes, preferably with pads of cotton soaked in witch hazel over the eyes, maintaining the water temperature as necessary.

Breathing

The simple art of breathing almost deserves a chapter of its own. Breath is life—and to learn to regulate breathing is in effect to learn to control the life force. Each and every meditation exercise requires you to concentrate on breathing. Altering your breathing can literally alter your state of mind. In physical terms, the brain works on oxygen; the simple act of inhalation is nourishment. Exhalation of carbon dioxide expels waste from the body. Everything on earth breathes—humans, plants, animals. The universe itself can be said to breathe.

Breathing can relax you, distance you, and fuel you for physical activity. Controlled breathing controls stress and can boost the immune system, as well as help to overcome debilitating diseases like emphysema and asthma.

Controlled breathing exercises range from the yogic science called *pranayama* to the Chinese tradition of *qigong*. It may take some experimentation to find the breathing method that is right for you—one that will help you attain a feeling of centeredness, relaxation, and alignment with the rhythm of the universal breath.

For starters though, try this simple exercise: Stand up straight with your feet together and eyes forward. Inhale in a long slow breath, lifting your arms from your sides to high above your head in a long, slow stretch. When you've reached the top, turn palms down and allow your arms to float gently back to your sides as you exhale. Repeat eight times a day to increase the body's resistance to stress and boost immunity.

Chakras

The word *chakra* is taken from the Sanskrit word for wheel. The seven main chakras are thought to be the energy centers of the body—"wheels" of vibration—

ruling both physical and nonphysical functions. Some esoteric literature defines as many as twelve chakras, while others, defining the chakra centers into major and minor classifications, identify as many as three hundred and sixty. The proper opening of specific chakra centers are believed to put the individual in alignment with both the self and the larger universe, making him or her more receptive to spiritual information, which in turn results in better health and increased awareness.

Corresponding with specific locations along the spine and the central nervous system, the seven main chakras are believed to channel the life force from the universe. There are significant differences between eastern and western views of the chakras, but under the western system, the seven chakra centers are generally defined as follows:

The testicles or ovaries represents the first or root chakra.
The spleen and adrenals represent the second chakra.
The abdomen represents the third or stomach chakra.
The heart represents the fourth or heart chakra.
The thyroid represents the fifth or throat chakra.
The pituitary represents the sixth or brow chakra.
The pineal represents the seventh or crown chakra.

In addition, the seven chakras are thought to have an association with a specific planet, as follows: Pluto rules the first chakra, Mars rules the second, Mercury rules the third, the Sun rules the fourth, Venus rules the fifth, Neptune rules the sixth, and Uranus rules the seventh or crown chakra.

It is believed that the four lower chakras are governed by the four elements. Earth rules the root chakra and is at the lowest level of vibration. The right amount of energy here will impart a sense of stability. Too much energy centered here or a blockage of earth energy will make a person slow to change, fearful, and timid. Not enough energy will make a person feel ungrounded and indecisive.

The second chakra is ruled by the element of water. Too much energy here and you will feel hypersensitive, and unable to separate your own feelings from those of other people. Too little energy here and you will feel isolated—"dried up." The right amount of energy will give the person a sense of literally "going with the flow."

The third chakra is ruled by the element of fire. An important area for healing, it has to do with how energy is absorbed and balanced. Such things as eating disorders are due to an imbalance or blockage in the third chakra.

The fourth chakra is ruled by the element of air. It relates to objectivity and the ability to conceputalize. Too much energy here will make a person compulsive and anxious. Too little and the person will become out of touch.

With a little practice you will be able to sense the quality of energy in both your own and other people's chakras. Remember, the idea when dealing with chakras is to establish of sense of the flow of energy from one point to another. When energy is blocked, flow is blocked also. Therefore, in opening and aligning the seven chakra points, the elemental rulers should be taken into account, as well as the element governing the planetary ruler of a particular chakra point, particularly when a planet is shown to be badly aspected in the natal chart.

Candle Burning

Candle burning has long been associated with alternative healing, magic, and self-hypnotic procedures and practice, probably because of a candle flame's ability to focus the individual's attention, often to the exclusion of any other outside influence or distraction. For purposes of this volume, the use of candles is highly recommended in healing ritual, especially ones that are scented or colored to correspond with the elemental profile of the individual involved. Candlelight itself is pleasant and soothing to the eye and its healing properties can only be enhanced by appealing to the other senses.

Color Therapy or Chromotherapy

Chromotherapists believe that certain energies are augmented, balanced, or altered by exposing the seven chakra points to the seven colors of the spectrum. Some therapists expand the discipline to include the seven whole tones of the scale as corresponding to the seven colors and therefore to the chakra points. The appeal of chromotherapy is naturally sensual in origin, being quite obviously related to sight, yet its therapeutic value is perhaps easier to grasp if one thinks of color simply as a kind of light. And if light can be thought of as energy, the use of specific colors to align and heal the energy centers of the individual becomes quite easy to understand.

Recent scientific experiments have documented the various effects of different colors on the mind and emotions; similar beneficial effects of color on the physical form can also be expected. The human body, like all other life forms and organisms on earth, is quite capable of selecting from the spectrum of sunlight just which kinds of light it requires.

Color therapy then, can be thought of as a way to "boost" the body's natural resources and healing abilities in a noninvasive way.

The specific healing properties of color are described as follows:

Red: Stimulant, energizing, irritant. Red is thought to be the color associated with the first chakra and is believed useful in healing sexual dysfunction. Also thought to be the primary stimulant of the five senses and the liver, and to have beneficial effects upon the circulatory system.

Orange: Attuned with the second chakra, orange is believed primarily to be a respiratory stimulant, but is especially useful in any kind of congestion or blockage including constipation, fluid collection in the joints in diseases like arthritis, and menstrual disorders.

Yellow: Relates to the third chakra, believed to be the center of our emotions—the gut feeling. Used to strengthen the nervous system, increase alertness and mental faculty, and increase positive emotional reactions.

Green: Associated with the fourth chakra, green is considered the ideal healing color for balance, relaxation, and general healing purposes.

Blue: Linked with the fifth, or throat, chakra, blue is considered especially effective for cooling and antiseptic purposes, for alleviating pain, and for opening the individual to greater degrees of spiritual influence generally.

Indigo: Associated with the pituitary gland and the third eye, indigo awakens inner knowing and raises the level of vibration. Also considered beneficial in treating the eyes, ears, and sinus, and thought to have great influence upon the nervous system.

Violet: It is said that Leonardo da Vinci meditated under violet rays falling from a stained-glass window. The most highly spiritually charged of the healing lights, violet can prove too stimulating for some people. Linked with the crown chakra, violet is considered effective in treating neurological problems, migraines, and mental illness.

A simple experiment to determine whether or not you as an individual respond well to color therapy is to attach a color gel (easily purchased in an art-supply store) to a lamp or sunny window, and stand or sit in the rays of the resulting light for ten minutes. If you prefer, direct the colored rays to a specific part of the body for healing. Carefully note the results and experiment with different colored filters to see which works best for you and corresponds most compatibly with your own natural energy.

Crystals and Gemstones

Though crystals and gemstones were probably coveted in prehistory more for their visual appeal than their talismanic and healing value, the practice of using crystals and gems to channel universal energy and focus it for individual purposes is very old indeed. The lost civilization of Atlantis was believed to have fallen due in part to the misuse of crystal energy.

Although much of the original knowledge concerning crystals and gemstones has been lost to us, the premise behind the modern use of crystals is quite simple: All such stones have a crystalline structure and composition and as such are able to draw, collect, focus, and emit energy. This basic principle now operates throughout our everyday physical existence—quartz crystals provide power for watches and computer chips. A crystal, set in an energy field, will draw energy from that field—when pressure is applied to crystals they, in turn, emit measurable amounts of energy. Clearly there are physical laws by which crystal energy operates, but they have yet to be adequately defined. If you accept that energy is real—even though it is not always visible to the naked eye—and that the human body emits energy, then you can also accept that a person's energy field can be affected, for better or for worse, by coming in contact with other known fields of energy.

To accept the power and potential of crystals and gems, one has only to accept that both physical and spiritual life is governed by laws we have yet to fully understand or define.

The astrological signs have long been associated with birthstones and gems. One theory of crystal knowledge states that traditional birthstones are best used for the affairs of everyday life, while the use of gemstones associated with the astrological signs are more suited to activities like enhancing spiritual awareness. From the point of elemental analysis of the individual chart, however, it becomes possible to select from a sizable group of crystals and stones associated with the vibrational qualities of your ruling-element group. Take care when selecting a crystal for healing purposes that it is of natural rather than synthetic origin. The popularity of crystals has led to something of a boom in the manufacture and sale of synthetic stones, and while some of the laboratory-produced stones are quite beautiful, they simply do not carry the same energy level as those found in nature. Most urban areas can now boast of at least one reputable rock and mineral shop, and the dealers are usually a fine source of information about the field. Please refer to the Crystal Keys, beginning on page 199, and suggestions for the use of crystals throughout later chapters.

A final introductory word about crystals and elemental work is only that when using them Fire- and Earth-ruled personalities will respond more readily to crystals in their natural form, simply because Fire and Earth are the elements that combined to make the stones in the first place. Water people might do well to take their crystal healing in another form—gem elixirs, for example, see page 112. While Air-ruled personalities, with their highly strung nervous systems, can be especially responsive to a crystal's vibrational charge, they should approach crystal use with a measure of caution—hanging a healing crystal in a window or keeping an attractive geode on the nightstand might prove ultimately more effective for this personality than keeping in actual, constant physical contact with a stone, as in the form of jewelry, for example. For more detailed information, see Crystal Keys beginning on page 199.

Herb and Flower Therapies

Again, the use of flowers and herbs for both spiritual and physical healing is a practice almost as old as mankind. Though herb, flower, and aroma therapies are all intimately linked, each has developed into a specialty of its own—the famous Bach flower remedies being only one example. For the purposes of this book, however, herb and flower therapies will not be considered separately, since both involve much the same practices, i.e., the use of fresh or dried bouquets in the environment, the ingestion of teas, salads, and infusions, or the applications of packs and poultices for specific ailments. Herbalism can employ any part of the plant: root, stem, leaves, flowers, or fruit. Any element group can benefit from herb and flower therapies, though Water and Earth most particularly so. Fire-ruled personalities might want to consider including in the herbal aspect of their healing rituals some form of herbal incense, cooked or burned herbs, while Air types should consider especially the use of aromatics, vapors, and dried herbs and flowers. General directions for the preparation of both herbal infusions and decoctions are included below. Please refer to the individual chapters for specific suggestions regarding herbs and healing.

Herbal Infusion

An infusion is a beverage made as a tea is made—pouring boiling water over herbs and allowing the mixture to steep, in order to extract the plant's natural benefits. The water should be at a rolling boil when used, then the mixture should steep and cool to drinking temperature or longer before straining. The short exposure to heat helps to guard against the loss of volatile elements. The usual proportions for an herbal infusion made in this way are one cup of water for every ounce of dried herbs or two ounces of fresh.

Herbal Decoction

The decoction method of preparation is used when you wish to extract minerals and essences from hard materials like bark and roots. Add 1 ounce of plant material to 2 cups of cold water; bring to a boil over medium heat and boil gently for 10 minutes. Remove from heat, cover, and cool. Strain and use as desired.

Energizing Rosemary Bath

Of the herb rosemary, the famous seventeenth-century herbalist John Gerard said: "It comforteth the brain, the memorie, the inward senses and comforteth the heart and maketh it merrie." Rosemary is a wonderful all-around tonic herb, whose best properties can be readily absorbed through the skin in the form of a warm bath. Steep 2 ounces dried rosemary leaves in one pint boiling water for 10 minutes. Add to the bath to energize the metabolism, stimulate circulation, and aid the digestion.

Homeopathy

In recent years, the term *homeopathy* has been expanded to include many so-called "natural" remedies, but in fact, the practice of homeopathy is based upon the idea that like cures like—that minute portions of a substance will stimulate the body's natural defenses and recuperative powers to effect a cure for whatever ails you. Instead of the use of a cough suppressant, for example, a homeopath will administer a small amount of a substance that would ordinarily trigger a cough, in the belief that such medicine will "jump start" the body's immune system. Homeopaths generally confine themselves to "natural" substances like herbal extracts, but they can also use amounts of equally natural, but lethal, substances in their pharmacopoeia—snake venom, for example. Since the amounts of any substance administered as a homeopathic remedy are so small and so diluted, question has arisen both with traditional and non-traditional healers as to whether such remedies do any good at all, or if their effectiveness is not in fact the result of a placebo effect. Yet, at the same time, it has become increasingly documented that the mind indeed affects the body. If you happen to believe a homeopathic remedy will cure your headache, it doesn't have to be scientifically proven when your headache goes away as a result of taking that medication. Use homeopathy as you would any of the treatments included in this book, no matter what your particular elemental profile. If you find it cures your headache, fine. Just don't expect homeopathy to cure a brain tumor. If for any reason you suspect a serious medical condition, use your own good sense and consult a physician, and continue to use the methods contained in this book to help and augment traditional medicine, not as a substitute for it.

Massage

Therapeutic massage has enjoyed a huge surge in popularity in the 1990s as evidenced by the rise of such retail chains as The Great American Backrub. Massage can improve circulation, loosen tight muscles and connective tissue, increase the supply of nutrients like oxygen in the bloodstream, and help the body rid itself of metabolic waste. From the healing perspective, all of this helps the body to heal itself and awaken both physical and spiritual receptors that have been deadened by chronic tension.

Beyond that, however, is the simple fact that the act of massage incorporates a mysterious human factor: Few things are more healing than the touch of another human being. Whether massage does indeed involve the actual transfer of energy from one person to another in a form of laying on of hands is not known, but is certainly probable.

Both eastern and western traditions of massage offer a wide range of options, ranging from pressure points to neuromuscular reeducation. Massage therapies include shiatsu, rolfing, Swedish, reflexology, sports massage and even self massage, to name a few. When divided into basic types a massage will fall into one of the following categories: Pressure points, muscular, and those involving connective tissue. Most professional massage therapists will combine the basic massage types into a unique massage style.

Different elemental types will respond more favorably to specific types of massage than others, so refer to the following chapters for specific suggestions on which type of massage will be most appropriate for you. Do remember, though, that when seeking a professional massage therapist, the object here—as with all of the healing therapies included in this volume—is pleasure, not pain. No massage should be painful—massage is designed to ease pain and stress, not create it.

Meditation

Meditation, simply defined, is the exercise of turning one's focus inward, thereby gaining distance, perspective, and, ideally, enlightenment. There is a huge range of meditation types and styles, but again, meditation exercises will usually fall into one of two categories: concentrative and mindfulness meditations.

Concentrative meditation requires the focusing of the individual's attention upon some activity or object such as a candle flame, picture, one's breathing, or the repetition of a keyword or mantra.

Mindfulness meditation is somewhat more sophisticated in that one's mind is in effect "allowed" to wander in the meditative state, but the practitioner perceives thoughts, feelings, and sensations in a state of heightened awareness.

What any meditation requires of us is that we "turn off" or "tune out" the outside world, in the interest of greater awareness of the inner, invisible realm, ideally resulting in a greater centering and uniting of body, mind, and spirit. It is believed that meditation can give us greater awareness, increased psychic ability, and what might best be described as a sense of spiritual "belonging"—that is, a sense of our identity in the larger universe.

What has been scientifically proven is that regular meditation has a significant effect on the body, including lowered blood pressure, improved immunity, and reduced anxiety.

The four elemental types will, as always, respond to various styles of meditation differently. The Air type, for example, would do well to choose a method that emphasizes breathing techniques; Earth types do well by focusing on some material object such as a candle flame as an approach to a meditative state.

Please refer to the specific suggestions and exercises for your elemental type in later chapters. And remember that meditation is a skill that can be learned. But, like any skill, it must be practiced regularly in order for you to become truly proficient. It is highly recommended that you set aside twenty minutes every day for meditation. Your individual approach might be something as simple as making the promise to yourself to spend those minutes in the pleasure of your own company, thinking your own thoughts. Or you might find that meditation isn't really useful for you unless you draw the shades, light the incense, and assume the lotus position. Whatever your individual inclinations, it is important that you experiment with different styles until you find one that's right for you.

Do be aware, though, that as useful as meditation can be, it is not magic. Very little will be gained from meditation if you approach it with the attitude that twenty minutes a day is going to completely remove stress from your life, or that you will find all the answers to life's conundrums in meditation. Asking for the answers is *prayer*. Meditation is not asking—it is *listening*.

One final suggestion to facilitate meditation is to set aside time during the day or night that is as close as possible to the time you were born. Obviously this is going to be easier for some people than others, but, at any rate, it is useful and appropriate to meditate every day and at the same time every day.

Music and Sound Therapy

Music therapy is an incredibly flexible tool for strengthening the mind, body, and spirit, and traditional medicine is now embracing the concept in everything from headphones at the dentist's office to the inclusion of formal music therapy classes in medical schools all over the country.

At is simplest, music therapy is what happens when a baby is soothed by its mother's soft lullabye; at its most esoteric, the theory of music therapy purports that each of the chakra points are activated by the seven whole notes of the musical scale by virtue of a vibrational response, just as they are in color therapy.

What we do know is that musical sounds, when they reach the brain, trigger positive changes in the immune, endocrine, and central nervous systems. Music has been seen to reduce anxiety, improve relaxation, and even to help learning disabled and head-injured patients recover basic movement and memory skills.

Basically music therapy can be explained in terms of its components—key, rhythm, and harmonics. Consider that every human being can be said to fluctuate in "major" and "minor" moods, or keys. Minor keys encourage us to be subjective and personal—to turn inward. Major keys create or enhance the urge to be outgoing, motivated, and creative. Certain rhythms can energize and motivate the physical form, as in martial marches or the trance-like dances incurred by people in certain native cultures. Harmonics are said to awaken the spiritual forces within us by virtue of their more complex vibrational affect, and most music therapists recommend the regular inclusion of music works that are characterized by stringed instruments like violins, since the sounds produced by such instruments operate at a frequency comparable to the human voice.

Obviously personal taste is crucial in selecting music for inclusion in your own healing and wellness programs. However, a few general guidelines are appropriate here. Below is a list of musical keys as they correspond to the seven energy centers in the body.

From the elemental standpoint, Water responds well to music in minor keys or tones, Earth to that written in major tones. Fire will respond well to the quarter-toned music of India while Air, with its emphasis on mental development, might consider exploring new age or Oriental music utilizing one-third tones.

Yet, if you don't know a quarter from a half note, or have the slightest notion of where to find Middle C, don't despair. The use of music therapy in your healing

Chakra	Musical Key	Color	Planet
First Chakra	C	Red	Pluto
Second Chakra	D	Orange	Mars
Third Chakra	E	Yellow	Mercury
Fourth Chakra	F	Green	Sun
Fifth Chakra	G	Blue	Venus
Sixth Chakra	A	Indigo	Neptune
Seventh Chakra	B	Violet	Uranus

program doesn't require anything by way of a musical gift or even a "good ear." Choose music you like to accompany your healing exercises. Some musical therapists recommend Baroque music as the best for healing, due to the heavy use of string and wind instruments, like the harpsichord, violin, and flute. Bach's *Brandenburg Concerti* or Vivaldi's *Four Seasons* are both excellent choices and available everywhere. Another option would be to explore the wealth of New Age recordings that are designed and advertised to aid healing and meditation. In choosing your musical selections, remember that quiet instrumental music is best. Some therapists recommend selecting music that is at or below your own heart rate—usually about sixty beats per minute. Perhaps most important, though, is that your music is pleasing, that it does for you what music does best—lifts you out of yourself, elevates your thoughts and spirit, and reminds your soul of its true nature. By adding music to your meditative and healing regime you can quite effectively "fine-tune" the instrument of self through music's healing vibration.

Pyramids

The use of pyramids and pyramid power has enjoyed a huge surge of popularity in the last ten years or so, but few people are aware of the history or origins of the pyramid, save for a vague general association with Ancient Egypt. Many mystic and occult scholars, however, believe that the use of pyramids in Egypt was in fact part of a larger body of ancient knowledge imparted from the lost civilizations of Atlantis and Lemuria.

The ancients were believed to have knowledge of how geometric shapes affected health and spirituality. It was thought that meditating upon—or exposure to—certain shapes could heal both the body and the mind and could affect the growth of individual consciousness. Of the different shapes used, the pyramid and the mandala were the most popular. From information obtained from channeled spiritual communication, it is believed that ancient pyramids were built from crystalline materials and that the combination of energy-drawing shape as manifested in the pyramid, combined with the use of crystalline structures in these lost civilizations, may have in fact contributed to their destruction, due to the resulting disturbance in the earth's energy fields from such great concentration in one or two spots.

Basically, what pyramids do is amplify the natural energies of that which is placed inside them. For healing purposes, the effectiveness of crystals, personal talismans, herbal oils, teas, and essences are thought to be enhanced when placed under a pyramidal structure. Power pyramids can be constructed of just about anything, but it is recommended that they be made of natural materials. Gold, silver, and copper sheeting are best, but a pyramid can also be constructed in skeletal form using any kind of wood. The placement of quartz crystals at the midpoint of each side helps to enhance the structure's power, as does a magnet or loadstone placed inside. One point of the pyramid should face due north; and when placing objects underneath—or meditating beneath—a pyramid, it is best done in the morning when the life force is thought to be strongest.

Visualization

Visualization techniques can be of great benefit both in spiritual and physical healing, but the success of visualization depends in large portion on the ability of the individual to visualize—to create detailed, vivid pictures of the object or situation he or she wishes to effect. But even if you don't conceive of yourself as highly visual, imagery can work for you. The average person has up to three thousand random images flit through their mind every day. Visualization can give you a way to shape those images to achieve a desired result. Researchers are beginning to examine the possibility that patients can have a direct impact on their immune systems, on pain, and on general wellness with highly encouraging results.

If you plan to incorporate visualization, or guided imagery as it is sometimes called, into your personal healing program, you will probably achieve better results at the outset if the image you choose is highly emotionally charged. If you suffer from chronic pain, for example, it may not do much for you to imagine the pain is a baseball that you hit out of the stadium. On the other hand, if you regularly call up an image of yourself as happy, pain free, and involved in some favorite activity like dancing, you may see results.

Below are two simple exercises in visualization that can work for anyone, any time, anywhere. Designed to relieve stress, they can also give you a good indication of your own capacities for creating productive mental images.

> Close your eyes and call up a mental picture of the ocean. Watch the waves rolling into shore. See yourself lying comfortably on the shore. Watch as the water rolls over your body—feet, hips, chest— all the way up to your neck. As each wave draws back, feel the water pulling tension away from your body.

> Close your eyes and imagine yourself blowing up a balloon. Feel yourself blowing your stress into that balloon with each exhalation. Blow the tension out of your body. See the balloon grow bigger as you fill it with all your expelled stress and negativity. Imagine the balloon bursting, harmlessly evaporating your tension and stress into the atmosphere.

The Earth Personality

THE ELEMENT OF EARTH HAS BEEN MUCH MALIGNED IN some estoeric literature, having been reported in various accounts as being slow, lethargic, stubborn or operating at the "lowest" level of spiritual vibration. Earth people are also said to be calculating, mired in tradition, insensitive, and hopelessly limited by their bonds to the physical universe—as having a sort of "show me" perspective even when dealing with things ephemeral and invisible. Much of this perspective on Earth can be put in context when it is remembered that up until quite recently, western thought concerned itself with nature only as a force to be conquered. The earth at its best was to be plundered, at its worst, to be feared. Obviously, the element Earth has gotten something of a "bad rap" in many discussions and interpretations.

When it comes to the run of occult and New Age thought, then, it is easy to see why Earth-ruled people seem to be less than responsive to certain belief systems and alternative healing therapies, having already been rather effectively labeled as what might be called the spiritual stepchildren of the cosmos.

Yet nothing could be further from the truth. When it comes to reaching the soul and spirit through the five senses—when it comes to healing through something as simple as giving the body pleasure, perhaps no element is better equipped to benefit from that thing we call sensual healing than the Earth-ruled.

These people excel in the realm of the senses. Earth people are the closest to and most at home on this planet. Many have a heightened sense of awareness given to them by their superior sensory abilities. The tangible pleasures of fresh, whole foods, fine music, subtle color, complex fragrance, and rich texture are never entirely lost on the Earth personality, and it is from these things that Earth gets nourishment.

Perhaps Earth people have gained a reputation for being grasping and materialistic because at some level they do indeed recognize that for them material things are the way to spiritual wholeness. They really can find God in the little things. They are attuned to the universal energy through form. In a very real way, Earth people derive their energy from the physical universe. They change as the earth itself changes, slowly. Earth has patience, self-reliance, persistence, and endurance.

They are the best equipped of any type to be able to identify and meet their own needs and, to some extent, the needs of others as well. Earth people are practical about life, but, perhaps more important, they also have a real sense of the spiritual value of creature comforts. They can make life comfortable for other people, too, if given the opportunity.

The Earth-ruled personality is capable of channeling the energy of the universe to manifest physical life. By and large, Earth people seek closeness to the life force in the form of growing things—children, pets, plants, or even growing businesses. They love to "build from the ground up"—it is how they nourish the energy field within. Without the opportunity to nurture in some fashion, Earth people become irritable and depleted more easily than might seem possible for what is generally a hardy physical type.

Nonetheless, these are people who are, by and large, comfortable within their own bodies. They understand themselves as physical beings dwelling within a physical universe that operates by predictable (if not always fully understood) physical laws.

To understand better how to heal the Earth type, it helps to understand first how this personality deals with conflict, since it is to a large extent conflict that gives rise to a need for healing in the first place.

Earth rarely creates conflict; because they take challenge so seriously, they rarely go out in search of it, or indeed of confrontation of any kind. When conflict does arise, however, the Earth person absorbs it slowly, by degrees. They are slow to anger, yet capable of astonishing force when the need arises. Think of a lazy summer day exploding into a destructive tornado, a sleepy winter afternoon giving way to a howling blizzard. The storms seem to come without warning, but in fact they come because there has been a build-up in the atmosphere, creating a need for release.

So, too, with the Earth person. More than any other group, they are apt to accumulate tension and toxicity in the psyche and in the physical body, sometimes without visible effect or even their being aware of it. Earth people are not, as has been so frequently reported, insensitive—it is simply that with their great natural strength they are capable of storing up without complaint the hurts, the slights, the million little sensory assaults of modern life to a point that others might find unendurable. Seen another way, the Earth personality is so sensorily aware that too much negative input through the senses—i.e., bad food; the smell in the subway; the ugliness of a grey urban landscape, etc.—will eventually lead to a shutting down or closing off of the more sensitive aspects of Earth's personality as they concern themselves with the more obvious aspects of endurance and survival.

Healing, for this type, should address itself to enabling the earth person to let go of accumulated tension, buried conflicts and environmental stress before the storm begins to blow. Once their energy field is cleared of such accumulations, most Earth types will reveal themselves to be capable of astonishing perception and real spirituality. The Polynesian word for "psychic" is literally translated as "to observe the patterns of time." And that is a very accurate description of how the spiritual nature of Earth becomes manifest. They know, as the earth itself knows—the patterns of time.

Specifically, Earth responds beautifully to healing techniques that employ things that are of the earth. Herbs and crystals are the obvious choices here, but anything that involves the tangible, rather than intangible, will evoke a greater and faster response from the Earth-ruled personality than a method employing too much in the way of abstraction. The Earth person should take special note of the simple fact that many, if not most, ailments are not anything more or less than very obvious physical manifestations of inner states of being, and that those connections are very logical by nature.

Shoulder pain, for example, can be traced to a feeling of being overburdened, of carrying the "weight of the world." Arthritis and joint pain (particular afflictions of the Earth personality) can be related to a literal lack of flexibility in one's attitudes and beliefs. Finally, remember that Earth loves and has a great need for physical beauty in their homes, offices, and general environment. Though the Earth personality may not give voice or even be consciously aware of a highly developed sense of the aesthetic, something as simple as a well placed vase of flowers or an attractive geode can do much to soothe and heal the soul of misunderstood Earth.

The Earth/Fire Personality

This personality can best be characterized by a single word—drive. They simply have more of it than any other pure type or combination-type personality. Here the endurance of earth gives power to the self-expressive needs of fire. Earth gives fire patience and fire gives earth faith. Like the popular commercial character, the Earth/Fire personality keeps "going and going and going and . . . " They are life's marathoners, able to conserve and direct their sometimes formidable vitality toward a desired end. Ambitious in the extreme, Earth/Fire is the ultimate self-starter. Though they may not be smarter or more talented or luckier than anybody else, they get what they want simply because they want it more than anyone else.

Though Fire by itself needs the adulation and approval of others, Earth/Fire tends to be something of a loner. This is due in part at least to their tendency to sidestep the rules that govern more conventional lives, believing that it is easier to get forgiveness afterwards than it is to get permission beforehand.

Earth/Fire is as subtle as a Mack truck and there is a danger of them falling prey to an excess of sensory input and a love of sensationalism for its own sake. You won't find many real drug addicts or alcoholics here, but their habits of consumption are such that you may think so. You may also find overeaters, the oversexed, and the compulsive thrill seeker, though they are, by and large, possessed of such enormous physical resources that they will probably not do themselves much damage in the long run.

Are they insensitive? Well, more timid souls trying to get the number of that truck might have a different tale to tell, but Earth/Fire is not innately insensitive. They are, however, so utterly self-reliant it can sometimes seem as though the rest of the population is somehow incidental. They don't need much in the way of support, comfort, or shoulders to weep on, and don't really understand why other people do.

But amazingly enough, Earth/Fire has the best chance at and capacity for finding real love—passionate, sexual, stable, boundless, generous, eternal-type love, and it might very well be the promise of love that leads them to seek greater attunement with the larger cosmos and alignment with a more universal rather than personal energy in the form of healing. As the object of Earth/Fire's desire, you could do worse. Catch one on their way to the top and build an empire together.

The trick, of course, is to get their attention.

The Earth/Air Personality

The key word for this type is logic. Relentless, efficient, and admittedly sometimes humorless logic. Earth/Air is a configuration that takes itself and the rest of the world quite seriously and rarely indulges itself in things like fundamental relaxation.

Yet it may be surprising to learn that there is often very little in the way of real inner conflict within the Earth/Air personality, though these elements themselves are traditionally thought of as noncomplementary. Consider that the Earth signs—Capricorn, Taurus, and Virgo—and the Air signs—Gemini, Libra, and Aquarius—share some of the same planetary rulers, Venus and Mercury. Thus the Earth/Air energy combination is seen as more innately functional than not, due to the fact that their common planetary rulers approach life in much the same way, with many of the same priorities.

Earth/Air makes perhaps the best business person in the elemental system, given their innate abilities to access the world of ideas and manifest those ideas in practical ways. They are wonderful problem solvers and administrators, and can show an amazingly innovative approach to getting things done. They can be at home in a bureaucratic or even a diplomatic setting, where areas like detail, form, and protocol figure largely into their responsibilities.

They do best, however, when their business responsibilities are kept quite separate from their personal lives, simply because Earth/Air is often just not very good at the more intimate, personal side of life. They are prone to worrying over real or imagined inadequacies, fears of intimacy, and at its most extreme, Earth/Air will show a complete withdrawal from the illogical, unmanageable, and unpredictable world of human relationships; surround themselves with things rather than people; and direct their more nurturing energies toward things like African violets or a bevy of cats. Yes, you will find many "old maids," and "confirmed bachelors" with this configuration, as they are extremely reluctant to adjust their lifestyles to accommodate others.

Sensual healing can be ideal for this type as it can allow them access to pleasant feelings and emotions in safe and controlled circumstances. No naked bodyrubs with heated oils for this group, though. But a vial of refreshing citrus oil to clear the mind and a nice cup of chamomile tea might do nicely, thank you. Relaxation methods that are methodical and progressive, working with specific muscle groups will find greater response here than a vague set of directives for allowing one's mind to wander freely over the vast expanse of the cosmos. Wandering in almost any form is bound to make these people a bit nervous. While the Earth/Air combination is sometimes seen as controlling, it is my own opinion that they are not so much interested in controlling or dominating others as they are rather genuinely terrified at the prospect of losing control over themselves. Obviously, it is not the same thing at all.

Healing that gently indulges without being emotionally overwhelming can impart to Earth/Air a sense of inner security they often lack, due to their fundamental distrust of the more unpredictable, irrational aspects of emotional life. Properly aligned, Earth and Air energies are capable of innovation, detachment, and truly brilliant administration. They have a wealth of ideas, formidable intelligence, and the simple stamina and practicality to see those ideas brought to fruition in the material world.

The Earth/Water Personality

These energies are inherently complementary and when rightly aligned, the personality will have a fine sense of practicality combined with a highly developed intuition. Water gives Earth sensitivity to others, while Earth gives Water security and a sense of groundedness. The Earth/Water personality runs deep; their insights into the human condition can be quite profound. Water serves to broaden Earth's sometimes narrow horizons through its connectedness to others, and imparts a sense of perspective. Earth in turn is nourished by Water's energy in a meaningful way.

A sense of the interconnectedness of all beings can find its highest expression in an Earth/Water type. They can be quite spiritual or religious in traditional ways, and self-sacrificing in the sense that they will work tirelessly for the benefit of others, usually in a very practical fashion. Ordinary saints can be found with this configuration—they understand in some fundamental way that the way to the spirit is through the body—that discourses on God and the soul don't mean very much to a body that is hungry or cold.

Perhaps part of Earth/Water's dedication to others is to be found in their own real need for security. They are often highly attached to their spouse or children, to having "enough" money, or to seeking to enhance a sense of self through material goods. Due to a highly developed sense of beauty, it is not unusual to find collectors with this elemental rulership. Yet such collections will never be idle accumulations of things. They will instead be made with an eye to their investment value as well as to beauty.

Healing the Earth/Water type through sensual means can certainly be effective, but often involves a few false starts as this type can be quite unconscious of their own motivations and needs. Personal comfort and physical security is essential, however, as they often manifest a number of previously unidentified fears when reaching a state of heightened awareness—fears that may be difficult to fully articulate, but that are intimately linked with a sense of their own survival.

At best the Earth/Water personality is well grounded, highly social, sophisticated in the ways of the world, and full of natural inner strength. At the worst, their groundedness becomes stodginess, their sociability manipulative, and their inner strength is manifest as frustrated obstinacy.

When Earth Energy Is Blocked

A blockage of Earth energy can manifest itself in a variety of ways in all of us, but can be especially detrimental to the health and well-being of the Earth-ruled personality. Simply put, a blockage of Earth energy is an accumulation of too much of that energy in the lower chakras. The activation and nourishment of the Earth personality's pleasure centers encourages the Earth energy to flow to the point where the sense of self is restored and proper alignment with the universal Earth energy is possible.

Below is a list of common physical and psychological complaints that are indicative of blocked Earth energy. Keep in mind that this list is equally useful for those lacking or weak in the Earth elements—there are many points of intersection and similar manifestations, but treatment and therapies will vary, depending upon the individual's elemental rulership. The therapies included in this chapter are suggested for Earth-ruled types primarily. Balancing or augmenting a lack of Earth energy is far different from unblocking or freeing an accumulation of pent-up Earth energy.

PHYSICAL

Colds
Constipation
Arthritis and inflammation of the joints
Acne or excessive oiliness in the skin
Muscle stiffness
Ankle or foot pain
Sciatica
Inability to lose weight
Kidney or bladder problems, especially stones
Poor circulation
Blood clots
Gout
Anemia
Poor digestion
Irregular menstruation
Prostate problems
Sexual dysfunction

PSYCHOLOGICAL

Preoccupation with material affairs, especially money
Fears for survival
Fear of change
A chronic sense of confusion
Depression
Sleeping too much
Inertia or a sense of futility
A tendency to take refuge in routine for its own sake
An overwhelming or inappropriate sense of respon-
    sibility (i.e., they can't get along without me)

An inability to articulate thoughts and feelings

Greed

A need to manipulate or control others

Defining personal strength as the ability to do without or engaging in destructive substitute gratification; i.e., not buying the new dress you wanted because you "don't need" or "can't afford it," then buying and eating a large anchovy pizza so the dress won't fit

"Penny-wise, pound foolish" behavior in general

Compulsive overindulgence in sex, food, drink, work, shopping, or gambling

Inability to nurture others

Earth and the Five Senses

It may seem utterly simplistic to say that, more than anything else, people with a preponderance of Earth energy need to get outside once in a while. But just because a thing is simple doesn't mean it isn't true. Earth nourishes its own energy by regular contact with the world of nature. They need to wriggle their bare toes in the mud, to get their hands dirty, to putter about in the garden at regular intervals. Urban Earthers who don't have much access to nature as we know it might consider scheduling regular pastoral vacations—even a short as a weekend—to places that will put them in greater contact with the smells, sights, and sounds of the natural world.

Scheduling those trips when the sun is in one of the Earth signs—Taurus, Virgo, or Capricorn—would prove most beneficial; barring that possibility, choose a time when the moon is in an Earth sign.

But none of us, most particularly Earth signs, can truly integrate body, mind, and spirit in a few short trips a year. In fact, Earth can be quite reluctant to depart from their usual routines for any reason at all. Yet, even the most dogged Earth soul can benefit enormously from a few simple noninvasive additions to their homes and life-styles in the form of pleasurable sensory input.

The Sense of Sight

More than anything else, the Earth personality responds to warm tones in the personal or work environment, especially red and umber. Straight brown and beiges might be appealing to Earthers, but should be augmented with warmer tones because of their energizing effect. Consider painting a room or even a single wall in a deep terra-cotta tone. A rich oriental carpet, replete with a variety of reds, could provide a centerpiece for an Earth room, and prove doubly satisfying due to the investment value of such pieces. Use a red light bulb in a single lamp, or a red lampshade of sufficient transparency to bathe the room in warm light.

Visually, consider a fine Rembrandt print incorporating reds and earth tones. Other choices might be the works of Velasquez, Vermeer, or Fernando Botero. Earth people tend to respond to portraits in particular and to realistic works in general, so stay away from any disturbing abstract or non-representational modern or post-modern works as they tend to prove unnerving to the Earth-ruled psyche.

Earth people should also make a concerted effort to wear the color red at every opportunity. Even if it is something as conservative as a red silk necktie or a pocket square, the effects of this color prove energizing to Earth and should be always incorporated in some fashion. One Earth-ruled woman I know never departed from the standard beige or blue business suits she wore to the office, but always indulged herself in red silk lingerie.

It cannot be stressed strongly enough that Earth people should make an effort to surround themselves with things of the earth—things that will provide regular visual cues to Earth energy. A bouquet of red roses or carnations arranged with sprays of eucalyptus and placed on the desk during a tough week at work will have a positive energizing effect, as will potted plants of almost any variety kept in the home or office. Naturally, pots of herbs specific to Earth energies are an excellent choice. See the chart on page 41. Remember that Earth-ruled personalities are at their best when growing something, even if all that it involves is watering a plant. Alternatively, decorative crystals or geodes can be effective, especially when placed on a sunny windowsill to attract and focus their energies. Refer to the Crystal Keys, beginning on page 199, for those gems and minerals specific to Earth vibration.

The Sense of Sound

Earth energy as manifest in the first chakra vibrates to the key of C major. Depending upon personal taste, Schubert's *March Militaire*, Holst's *The Planets*, and

J. S. Bach's *Brandenburg Concerto* in C major are all excellent choices. Earthers might also consider meditating to audio tapes and recordings of nature. Such recordings offer a huge range of choices—from birds singing and waves on the ocean to loons on a lake or a chorus of night sounds. Look for selections that you find relaxing and stimulating simultaneously. If native drum recordings appeal to you, go for it. If Celtic bagpipe music truly gets your blood up, use it.

Even if you have no ear or inclination for music at all, try accompanying your own meditations by tuning yourself to the key of C. Using a pitch pipe, find C and practice allowing yourself to duplicate the sound. Inhale deeply and as you exhale, sing the C. At first, stick with a simple Ahhh or Oooh sound. The important thing is to bring the sound up from the area of the first chakra, the base of the pelvis, and feel it rising up through your body and out of the top of your head. It will be easier at first if you keep one or both hands on top of your head to feel the vibration as you bring it forth. This exercise may take some practice, but it is highly beneficial. Get used to the sound of your own voice vibrating in tune with Earth energy, even if it makes you feel a little silly at first. Any exercise can seem silly until you get good at it and begin to see and feel its benefits.

The Sense of Taste

Earth-ruled personalities like to eat, no question about it. It is for these souls that the phrase "comfort food" was probably coined. They usually have sophisticated palates, though there is a tendency to poor dietary habits, due to their fondness for rich foods and sauces and the likelihood of excess protein intake. This is a personality that feels the need for a substantial "meat and potatoes" sort of diet. Additionally, Earthers can be prone to eating disorders of the binge-and-purge variety, or display a contemptuous disdain for "grazing" on such things as salad, fruits, and herbs.

Still, a few adjustments to the diet of the Earth-ruled personality can do much to heal body and soul. The judicious use of herbs can appeal to their culinary sense and talents, while the regular intake of greater amounts of non-fat carbohydrates and, yes, even chocolate can alleviate their tendency to depression and inertia.

Increased consumption of carbohydrates (including chocolate) encourage the production of tryptophane, a substance that, in turn, increases production of serotonin in the brain, resulting in a greater sense of general well-being.

In real terms, the Earth-ruled personality would do well to sit down to a plate of lightly-sauced pasta or indulge in the occasional chocolate truffle when they feel their energy to be at an especially low ebb. Earth types will also derive considerable pleasure and health benefits from the occasional glass of a good *digestif* such as Armagnac or a fine ruby port. While overindulgence is not encouraged, in moderation these liqueurs help control cholesterol, aid relaxation and the digestive process, particularly after a substantial, Earth-type meal.

Finally, the Earth-ruled personality can derive much in the way of satisfaction and an increased sense of well-being by experimenting with spicier cuisines—Mexican, Indian, and African dishes employing the use of seasonings like red pepper, chilies, and curries. Though the Earth-ruled may not be inclined to much in the way of experimentation, such cuisines tend to be lighter in their use of red meats and fats and richer in carbohydrates, while the fiery spices can do much to augment and encourage Earth energy. Please refer to the reference list on page 85, and the page following for recipes and further suggestions.

The Sense of Touch

A highly developed tactile sense characterizes many Earth-ruled personalities, and, practical as they are, most won't be content with Herculon when they can get velvet upholstery, nor with a kilim when they can roll around on something with a deep, plush pile. They won't settle for fiberfill pillows when they can have feather, nor should they. Earth is sensual, remember; they love the luxurious and equally love the luxury of touch. The closer they stick to natural textures, the more in harmony with their own energies they will be.

Think of settling down to meditate on a wooly sheepskin, or covered by a scarlet cashmere throw, and you may begin to get an idea of being at one with Earth. However politically incorrect it may be at the moment, Earthers just love fur. And silk, cotton, soft kidskin, and real leather, too. Natural fibers and materials are the key. The closer they are to the earth in the tactile sensations with which they surround themselves, the happier they are.

Earth people would do well in general to carry a small tiger's eye, both for its Earth-grounded energies and as a stone to touch and hold, off and on throughout the day, almost as one would a rosary or worry beads. A piece of carnelian would do equally well, and is purported to draw money—a plus for anyone, but especially for an Earth-ruled personality.

Additionally, this type responds best of all the elemental types to massage that employs the effleurage method of long strokes worked along the large muscle groups, together with vigorous muscle kneading. Earth types tend to be somewhat more heavily muscled than others, though heredity is obviously a factor. Effleurage helps to move the veins and to stimulate circulation, particularly when using a stimulating oil, scented with juniper, pine, or basil. Massage for the Earth-ruled should concentrate on the back—especially the lower back and the base of the spine, the principle location of the Earth-ruled chakra. Keep in mind, however, that when a massage is performed while the body is perspiring, as after vigorous exercise, or after a hot or steam bath, scented or essential oils will not readily be absorbed through the skin. While it will still smell pleasant, some of the beneficial qualities of the oil are apt to be lost.

The Sense of Smell

The Earth-ruled personality responds well to what might be called "heavier" scents in the form of herbal and essential oils, potpourris, and personally blended sachets. Though quality potpourris and sachets are still relatively easy to come by, especially when dealing with a reputable dealer (see appendix, page 217), I recommend the use of homemade herbal oils as described on page 42, because it is becoming increasingly difficult to obtain genuinely distilled essential oils. Synthetic or blended counterparts can be useless for healing on the one hand, and downright hazardous to your health on the other.

Even with a huge resurgence in the popularity of aromatherapy and the use of scent to activate and invigorate pleasure centers in the brain, many people are still a bit foggy as to just how to use scent in their own healing programs. The answer is simply to incorporate healing scents into your life-style in a way that is both useful and non-cumbersome. If your particular type of Earth-ruled personality wouldn't be caught dead reeking of essence of cypress, don't wear it in the form of a perfume. Instead, carry a vial of scented oil on your person and sniff it when you feel a need to augment your energy. If that seems too much to cope with, try scenting your immediate environment with a few drops of oil placed on a copper penny tucked away in a handy desk drawer. Alternatively, light a suitably scented candle at the end of a long day to revive your spirits; carry a small sachet in your purse or briefcase; or keep a few sprigs of one of the recommended herbs in your pocket or hanging from your rearview mirror.

Aromatherapies may be applied to specific Earth ailments as charted below, but for general tonic and healing purposes, the Earth-ruled should surround themselves with the scents of cedar, cypress, juniper, and pine. Cinnamon, vetivert, and clove are also good for Earth types—as are apple, patchouli, and vanilla. Earth types should find those scents invigorating to their natural energy; for relaxation purposes, however, such as a calming or purifying bath, choose from mimosa, oakmoss, lilac, and carnation. See the Monthly Healing Ritual for Earth (page 161) for additional suggestions.

Aroma Remedies for Some Common Earth Ailments

AILMENT	ESSENCE	FORM
Colds	Cinnamon, Clove, Eucalyptus	Tea or sachet
Cellulite	Cypress, Lemon, Lavender	Oil in bath
Constipation	Fennel, Tarragon	Seeds and leaves
Depression	Marjoram, Thyme	Sachet
Gout	Rosemary, Lavender	Poultice
PMS	Sage, Basil, Thyme	Fresh leaves
Rheumatism	Pine, Rosemary, Juniper	Oil in bath

Recipes for Earth Healing

Onion Tart

This is especially good for those suffering from menstrual disorders, oily skin, and rheumatic conditions. The onion is rich in vitamins and the sulfur in onions is good for the nervous system.

4 pounds of onions, peeled and sliced paper-thin
2 tablespoons butter or virgin olive oil
2 sprigs fresh rosemary
1 sprig fresh thyme
1 teaspoon caraway seeds
½ teaspoon sea salt
1 9-inch prepared uncooked pie pastry

Heat the butter or olive oil in a large skillet over medium heat. Add the onions and herbs, and simmer covered, stirring occasionally, until thoroughly cooked but not browned, about 15 minutes.

Arrange the onions evenly in the pastry, discarding the thyme and rosemary. Bake at 375 degrees for 25 minutes, or until the pastry is golden brown. Serve hot or cold.

Healing Pasta with Fresh Herbs

2 cups pasta, cooked
2 cloves garlic, crushed
1 tablespoon olive oil
Fresh basil, sage, thyme, and rosemary leaves,
to taste (the more the better)
Parmesan cheese
Fresh ground black pepper

Toss the above ingredients together and serve.

Earth Sachet

2 ounces sandlewood, powdered
5–6 drops patchouli oil
6 rosebuds, dried
2 ounces dried lavender flowers
4–5 cinnamon sticks, broken into pieces
2–3 nutmegs, whole (optional)
1–2 drops cypress oil (optional)

Blend powdered sandalwood with patchouli oil, dried rosebuds, lavender flowers, and broken cinnamon sticks. If desired, add nutmeg and cypress oil. Mix the ingredients thoroughly and place in sachet bags or potpourri bowls to be kept throughout the home.

Simmering Earth Potpourri

2 nutmegs, whole
3 cinnamon sticks
1 vanilla bean
½ ounce patchouli leaves
1–2 ounces pine needles
1 orange peel

In a small saucepan or potpourri simmerer, place whole nutmegs, cinnamon sticks, vanilla bean, patchouli leaves, and pine needles. Add orange peel and water to cover. Simmer as desired, at least one half hour, replenishing water as necessary.

Baths for Earth Healing

Calming Earth Bath

Add 3 drops oil of vetivert or 4 ounces vetivert decoction to running bath water, along with a handful of sea salt. Sprinkle the water with 2 ounces fresh red rose petals and as much fresh lavender as you desire.

Energizing Earth Bath

Add 3 drops oil of juniper or cypress, a handful of sea salt, 1 ounce of pure aloe vera gel, and the fresh peel of an orange to running bath water. Add the petals of red carnation or tint the water with a few drops red food coloring, if desired. Bathe by the light of a red candle.

Earth Breathing

This simple breathing exercise can be performed almost anywhere, any time. It is an excellent prelude to meditation. Inhale to a slow count of four. Hold for a count of twelve, exhale to a count of eight, concentrating on blowing the air out through an imaginary spot about three inches below your navel (the first chakra). Repeat four times or as desired.

Earth Affirmations

Simple affirmations of Earth energy, repeated to yourself—either in a state of meditation or simply on and off throughout the day—can do a lot for keeping yourself centered and your energy suitably aligned. Below are only a few samples. Try these to start and allow them to gradually evolve into your own personal power phrases.

> *I will survive.*
> *I inhale love; I exhale fear.*
> *I am able to express myself clearly, directly, and honestly.*
> *I draw my strength from the Earth beneath my feet.*
> *I attract to myself the universal bounty.*
> *The world is friend; the Earth is my mother.*
> *I am protected and free.*

The Water Personality

WATER PEOPLE ARE PERHAPS THE MOST DIFFICULT TO DEFINE
of any of the four elemental types, because they are so
varied in their natures—as different from one another
as a pond from an ocean, as a river from the falling rain.
The true Water type can be as harmless and happy as a
babbling brook one day—as destructive and dangerous
as a tidal wave the next.

Through the ages, Water souls have been described
as being everything from treacherous to poetic. Yet perhaps the true nature of the Water personality can be
defined in one word: "sensitivity." The Water type, more
than any other, is exquisitely sensitive to anything and
everything in the seen and unseen worlds. Water rules
the second chakra, the solar plexus, and Water types
are ruled themselves by nothing less than "gut" feelings—intuitions, hunches, and vibrations of all kinds.
True Water people are utterly connected to others by
virtue of their sensitivity. They pick up on the feelings,

signals, and vibrations—good and bad—of anything from lunar cycles to the secret anxiety of the man at the end of the bar as he awaits a blind date. This high degree of empathy can make Water wonderfully caring, deeply emotional, and highly psychic. It can also make for a personality that is difficult to understand, hard to pin down, and easily wounded.

Water energy, by virtue of its utter connectedness, is perhaps more in need of regular healing—through alignment and balance of body, mind, and spirit—than those with another rulership. As a form of energy, the element Water has the hardest time standing alone. While Earth energy can survive by virtue of its stead-fastness and practicality, or Air by escaping to the realms of the theoretical, i.e., retreating to an "ivory tower," Water's domain of pure emotion literally requires others (and other types of energy input) to become completely realized. In a sense, emotion has no identity of its own. After all, no one ever said, "I love, therefore I am." Yet Water energy, like love itself, endures all things, hopes all things and believes all things.

Only the Fire person requires others and their energy input in the way that Water does—primarily due to Fire's need to inspire and motivate, but Fire has at least the illusion of being grandly self-sufficient and self-reliant. Not so with sensitive Water souls—they are fully and sometimes quite frighteningly aware of their need for the constant emotional, vibrational, and intu-itive input that makes them what and who they are.

It is easy to see why they have sometimes gained a reputation for clinginess, manipulativeness, and dependency from interpreters who fail to make one fine distinction concerning the Watery nature. And that distinction is simply that there is a very real and crucial difference between being truly "dependent" and being "interdependent," a term that far more accurately describes the inner reality of the Water-ruled nature.

Perhaps it is their own awareness of this aspect of themselves that causes most Water types to cultivate what might be called a unique survival technique for wending their way through the world. Rather than involve themselves on deeper levels, many Water types will simply confine themselves to mirroring other people or their immediate environment, reflecting needs, desires, and aspects back in the same way one can find one's reflection in the glassy waters of a tranquil lake. Often, less sensitive and more egocentric types will convince themselves in very short order that they have discovered a true soulmate in the Water personality. Yet the mere narcissist is in for a rude awakening when the time comes for Water's true nature to reveal itself.

This tendency to "become what they see," feel, or touch is arguably Water's greatest strength, making them more truly adaptable, educable, and able to embrace a breadth of experience than even the Air personality. But great strength can also manifest as great weakness, making the Water type somewhat slow to form an identity separate from their loved ones, often easily dominated, and frequently loaded down with a variety of emotional baggage and stresses that may not even be of their own making—but rather consisting of other vibrations, bad moods, or emotional constructs that they picked up on and failed to properly release.

Water has a well-deserved reputation for moodiness. Being more emotional than any other types, it is certainly true that these sensitive souls have more than their share of ups and downs. But it should be remembered that moods in a Water personality are not mere performances, postures, or experiments. Though they will rarely bring the house down with a tantrum the way a Fire personality can, or indulge in a twenty-year quest for revenge like the Earth-ruled will, each change of these highly changeable tempers means something. Water moods are real—they are experienced fully. Water people feel more completely and intensely than any other personality type.

Yet a soul can easily drown in all those oceans of emotions, presenting the Water-ruled personality with a unique task in his or her quest for healing and wholeness. How can one experience and feel fully through the emotions and still maintain a measure of identity and security?

From the point of view of elemental and sensory healing, the answer can be found in the nature of water itself. Water moves on. Water takes for itself some of each of the other elements it encounters and allows itself to be altered by that experience, but always—ultimately moves on. Each wave from the ocean erodes some of the earth and then returns it. Water evaporates in its encounters with air, but returns to its true nature in the form of rain. Fire changes water into steam; steam rises, becomes air, condenses, and becomes water again.

Too many Water-ruled personalities have lost sight of that single aspect of their natures. In their quest for security and identity, they confine themselves to people or situations that have long ago ceased to be useful or nourishing, growing stagnant and depressed as a result. As brilliant as they can be at absorbing the thoughts, feelings, and vibrations of others, they can become curiously obsessed and weighted when they forget to release those vibrations. Some Water souls become sensationalists or addicts, believing that overloading themselves in one area will somehow deaden their overworked antennae in another. Still other Water souls will drift for years—lost and unfocused—seemingly unable to channel Water's energy in any kind of constructive fashion.

From both the sensual and spiritual standpoints, Water must learn to establish necessary boundaries by simply removing itself from the enormous amounts of sensory and intuitive vibration that Water encounters each day. Spending time alone, apart from the larger world, the Water personality can learn to channel its considerable energy and power. And Water does have power; make no mistake. It is power that belongs only to them and power they can learn to use if they simply protect themselves—intellectually, physically, and emotionally—from the demands of the world and learn to manage the intense sensitivity that defines them.

The Water-ruled personality is beautifully equipped to respond to healing, being naturally receptive and responsive to invisible energies, and already attuned to those energies in some fashion, whether consciously or not.

And while Water's insecurity may make it seem as though they cannot truly exist without others, it can also be said that nothing on this planet would exist without water—that no being can sustain itself for long without water's nourishment. It is only that the Water-ruled personality is so conscious of being needed by others, it often forgets to nourish itself.

The Water/Fire Personality

This is truly the most conflicted of all the Water configurations, including the Fire/Water personality as discussed on page 119. In the Fire-dominant type there is a stronger sense of self sufficiency and more natural optimism. Here, however, the individual can truly prove to be their own worst enemy. Water's natural tendency is to shyness, while Fire wants to assert itself. Water is never quite sure of what it wants, while Fire asserts its will.

This individual will be the first, therefore, to start an argument purely for the sake of stirring things up, and the first to feel wounded and victimized should they begin to lose that argument. Often difficult and unpredictable, these souls nevertheless have some significant advantages over the rest of us.

Brilliant humor of the wickedly irreverent, gallows type is here, along with remarkable loyalty and dedication. The ultimate "love me, love my dog" sensibility can be found in the Water/Fire personality. They often have truly astonishing memories, though that can include holding a real grudge against people or circumstances when they feel they have been wrongly used (which can be a lot of the time). Once you have overcome a well-defined defense system (and they will have one) they make wonderfully tolerant and astonishingly loyal friends. Perhaps it is because they are usually very aware of their own conflicts and imperfections—they tend not to be as hard on others as they are on themselves.

Healing presents a unique challenge for these souls. They are more prone to quite literally fizzle out when the going gets tough, Water tending to drown Fire's natural enthusiam with hesitancy and its passion with sentimentality. From a more purely psychological viewpoint, Water/Fire tends to a big ego accompanied by little or no self-esteem. They nevertheless respond wonderfully well to sensory input, being sensorily and emotionally oriented. It is never that the Water/Fire person can be said to be insensitive, rather that they tend to be too personally sensitive. Healing exercises and meditations that concentrate on taking this personality "out of himself" and putting their troubles, woes, and injuries in a larger, more universal context can prove transformative.

The Water/Earth Personality

Here we must examine the eternal opposition of the practical and impractical. Though these elements are essentially complementary, conflict can arise because Water "rules with the heart"—that is, by feeling and intuition, while Earth is governed by more practical impulses and considerations. Unlike the Earth/Water type discussed on page 73, there is more potential for conflict with Water as the dominant element, because they can sometimes prove to be the most serious threat to their own security interests. A Water/Earth type will find themselves continually torn between the sensitive, dreamy, emotional aspects of life and the practical, organized side. These individuals may fall into the trap of trying to organize and de-mystify their emotions through compulsive psychoanalysis, or give themselves over to their emotional lives completely—collapsing in tears at their unpaid bills.

At their best, however, these are downright comfortable people to be around. When the practical and poetic sides of existence are brought into alignment and these energies are allowed to complement, rather than conflict, the Water/Earth person is wonderfully sensual, artistically inclined or talented, and emotionally sensitive to others. They arguably make the best lovers in the world; have a natural inclination and fondness for sex of the more emotional kind; love creature comforts; and can be counted upon never to ignore or belittle that thing we call romance.

Yet Water and Earth do share a marked need for security, and so keep in mind that while this combination can make for magic, it can also make for mud. Apt to get mired in the deepest, longest, and widest ruts of all, healing should concentrate on a sense of progression or flow, utilizing the occasional infusion of Fire energy.

The Water/Air Personality

In its most evolved and aligned aspects, the Water/Air personality combines the intuition and sensitivity of Water with the intellectual and analytic powers of Air in what are generally considered to be brilliant and gifted observers of human nature. The movable, mutable nature of each decrees that they change—even metamorphosize—from time to time to really stay "fresh." They will probably change partners, careers, and locations with some frequency. There is sometimes an extreme tendency to self-invention and reinvention to the point of pathological lying, and there is likewise a certain tendency to believe that the rest of us are neither interested nor smart enough to catch them in one of their "stories."

They often prefer to "surf" the waves of existence, and are prone to the kind of disposition that is likely to remain the observer without ever allowing themselves to feel that they are participating fully.

Put another way, this configuration has a certain dislike and disdain for getting their hands dirty. They are wont to avoid what they perceive to be the treacheries of passion, though they remain very much interested in how passion works in other people. They can also—consciously or not—lead people on in an attempt to generate passion in order to observe it at close range, then be properly horrified to discover it directed at themselves.

They make brilliant writers and reporters; they can excel at pure investigative work. They are able to get to the heart of any matter or problem with great efficiency, yet their personal solutions to those problems might be equally lacking in heart as most Water/Air types are preoccupied to the point of neurosis with what they consider to be personal freedom.

Physically, the Water/Air personality is highly susceptible to environmental stress and blood pressure problems and—for all of their supposed distance and perspective—experience some very real conflicts between the mind and the emotions.

While they can do well in esoterics and sometimes even as ascetics, their essential restlessness craves variety and may lead them to a number of experiments with sensation for sensation's sake, though it is unlike them to become "addicted" to people, substances, or things in the more classic sense of the word.

The life of the Water/Air personality can be both weird and wonderful. They are the best natural eccentrics in the system. Creative, often brilliant, when properly aligned their energies can combine to produce works of great artistic merit, though these are more likely to be of the more avant-garde than classic variety.

Healing this soul involves anchoring it within the physical body in pleasurable and productive—not destructive—ways, for this personality can sometimes undertake destructive adventures or suffering in an attempt to make themselves "feel real."

So much of this soul's life is lived within that they must be encouraged to experience more of the physical world in aspects of tangible beauty, comfort, and encouragement. Regular gentle exercise like walking is helpful as is a diet providing adequate protein, since these are the souls who may quite easily "forget to eat," or nourish themselves on sugary snacks in an attempt to alleviate the bitter "nastiness" of ordinary life.

When Water Energy Is Blocked

The lack of alignment and attunement to Water energy can manifest itself in a variety of physical, psychological, and spiritual problems, the most obvious of which is that while these people may literally be drowning in a pool of their own emotions. They will have a great deal of fear and trouble when it comes to identifying their own feelings and those of other people. A person with blocked Water energy operates on a subconscious level a great deal of the time. This is especially true if the primary placement of the planets in the birth chart is in the southern or subconscious half, near the fourth house.

Blocked Water energy can also be indicated by chronic feelings of isolation and the inability to connect with others. In an attempt to be self-sufficient, those with an over-accumulation of Water energy will sometimes shut themselves down emotionally, while at the same time they will be curiously attached or dependent upon those who are able to express their own emotional natures. Alternatively, they may find themselves over-reacting to the slightest emotional stimulus, going to odd extremes in behavior, or be narcissistic or excessively self-absorbed.

Physically, blocked Water energy can express itself in obvious symptoms like water retention or unexplained weight gain, or in not so obvious things like excessive perspiration and night sweats, as the body and soul try to rid themselves of accumulated toxicity.

Below is a list of common problems afflicting those with blocked Water energy. While those lacking Water energy may experience some of the same problems, the treatments suggested later in this chapter are intended primarily for the Water-ruled personality.

PHYSICAL

Alcohol abuse
Bronchitis
Diarrhea
Diabetes
Lower back problems
Kidney problems
Excessive perspiration
Water retention or bloating
Weight gain
Liver and spleen problems

PSYCHOLOGICAL

Hypochondria
Chronic denial
Phobias
Nightmares
Compulsive self-sacrifice or martyr complex
Difficulties with timidity and dependence on others
Manic depression
Extremes in behavior or inappropriate emotional
    responses

Lack of control over, or inability to identify,
emotional responses in themselves and others
Inability to cope
Extreme impressionability
Lack of personal identity
Tendency to "smother" loved ones with excess
concern and emotion

Water and the Five Senses

The Water-ruled personality benefits enormously from
contact with water in all its myriad natural forms. A
walk by the ocean, lifting one's face to the falling rain, a
warm bath at the end of a long day, a serene row out to
the middle of the lake, a shower massage, or a trip to
the country to run barefoot through a babbling brook
are all ways in which Water can nourish and unblock
its own natural energies.

As always, healing exercises or trips should be
taken when the sun or moon is in a sign compatible
with the individual's energies—in this case a Water
sign; Cancer, Scorpio, or Pisces. Water people will
find that withdrawing from the workday world to
indulge themselves in sensory pleasure and healing
will be especially beneficial, since it is at these times
that emotional and psychic vibrations are especially
strong, and Water-ruled personalities may find themselves exhausted and depleted by an overabundance of
input and especially in need of nourishment for their
own personal energies.

The Sense of Sight

Despite the fact that many would believe that Water-ruled personalities are best inclined toward cool colors of blue, turquoise, and aqua, in fact, Water people do far better surrounded by the warmth of the orange and orange-yellow sector of the spectrum. Think of the bright hues of the islands against the blue of the Caribbean sea, the warm orange tile roofs of the fishing villages of the Mediterranean. Remember, Water is primarily the domain of the emotions—the second chakra point—and Water needs the warmth of orange both for healing and awareness. Beyond that, orange is cheerful, clear, and invigorating, all qualities much needed by sensitive Water souls.

In the home or work environment, orange can seem a rather difficult color to work into a decorating or fashion scheme, but it is not so. Tangerine and peach tones are both inviting and healing colors. They can add a sense of peace and prosperity to Water's sometimes disorganized surroundings. Such colors also complement and reflect skin tones and are easily worn for most people. A fluid length of a peach-colored silk chiffon scarf, a softly peach-colored dress shirt, or a briliant orange-rose boutonniere are all interesting possibilities for keeping orange's healing properties on your person. Orange encourages stability and has been said to activate the adrenals, to impart a greater sense of self-worth, and to aid in the assimilation of new ideas.

A bottle filled with orange-tinted water on a sunny windowsill will work subtle wonders on Water's state of mind, as will a painting or photograph of a fiery sunset or a field of orange poppies. Orange tulips, or better still orange or mock orange blossoms in a vase will provide an ineffable lift for the Water soul. Simplest of all, try a bright ceramic bowl of perfect oranges for both visual and aromatherapeutic healing.

Crystals might include stones like neutral citrine or fire opals worn as jewelry or carried as a personal amulet. Copper is also recommended for both its color and its ability to "draw" toxicity from the physical body.

The Sense of Sound

Most, if not all, Water-ruled personalities, if not gifted musically, have what is known in the vernacular as a "good ear." This is because Water personalties, on some level, are always "listening" in either the figurative or literal sense. Many are especially sensitive to harsh or unpleasant sounds in the environment, perhaps because all sounds are amplified "under water," and Water-ruled personalities thus perceive sound at greater levels of intensity. Most Water types will benefit from the regular use of some form of sound therapy.

The Water spirit as the ruler of the second chakra vibrates to the key of D major, and though sensitive Water types might find using a musical background too distracting for meditation, they will benefit from the healing qualities of music as they go about their daily routine.

Some excellent choices present themselves here, including Brahms' *Hungarian Dance No. 5*, Listz's *Hun-*

garian Rhapsodie No. 3 in D major, and Vivaldi's *Concerto for Flute and Orchestra in D Major*, Opus No. 10. For those moments when the Water-ruled personality feels the need for release in the form of a really good, uplifting sort of weeping session, try Tchaikovsky's *String Quartet in D Major*, most especially the *Andante Cantabile*. Music with a predominance of strings and woodwinds are excellent choices for Water people due to the fact that their vibratory range most closely approximates that of the human voice and connectedness is the key to unblocking an accumulation of Water energy.

Chanting or intoning the D major sound is also helpful for meditation. After finding the note on a pitch pipe, inhale and exhale the D major sound slowly in an "auummmm" sound until you feel your personal level of vibration attuning to the universal Water vibration and energy.

The Sense of Taste

Water-ruled personalties are subject to a variety of digestive upsets due to their extreme sensitivity. They are helped and invigorated by a diet rich in iron-rich greens, beta-carotene-rich vegetables like carrots and squash (due to their antioxidant properties), and lighter proteins in the form of legumes, fish, and chicken.

Most Water-ruled personalities have a great weakness for sugar as their delicate constitutions are easily depleted and prone to need the "lift" of sugary snacks or caffeine. While such snacks can be helpful under controlled circumstances, this tendency can just as easily lead to over-indulgence, bingeing, and the resulting weight gain. One Water-ruled personality I know never eats a regular dinner, but can sometimes be found late at night putting away a pint of ice cream or a package of cookies. In a very real sense, many Water people seek a sweetness from food that cannot always be found in life.

The tendency to overindulgence in sweets can be counteracted by the judicious use of herbs and herbal teas to the diet. A special emphasis on the increased consumption of fresh fruits and fruit juices will provide the Water-ruled personality with the sweetness they crave without so many of the unpleasant side effects of refined sugars. Sweet-hungry Water types should consider the occasional glass of an orange liqueur such as Grand Marnier as a substitute for that hot fudge sundae after dinner or at bedtime for increased relaxation.

Yes, eat oranges. Lots of them. Orange fasts one day a month are highly recommended to detoxify and invigorate the Water personality. The rich amounts of vitamin C that are found in oranges have also been shown to be especially useful in strengthening immune-system efficiency.

Specific culinary herbs recommended for the Water personality are chamomile, sage, yarrow, sweet marjoram, ginger, and angelica. Thyme, rosemary, basil, and hyssop are also very effective. Herbs should be taken primarily in fresh leaf or tea form with the addition of lemon and sweeteners as desired.

See the recipes and suggestions at the end of the chapter.

The Sense of Touch

From a purely tactile perspective, Water-ruled personalities will respond most readily to fabrics and textures that offer the qualities of fluidity, slipperiness, and cool smoothness. Satin, silk, and chiffon are excellent choices, though almost any finely woven fabric with what textile designers call "a good hand," that is, combining easy drape with lovely texture, is sure to appeal to the sensuous Water-ruled personality.

Water-ruled personalities are frequently cold. They seem to operate at a slightly lower body temperature than the rest of us and so are equally drawn to fabrics and textures that exude warmth, fuzziness, and thickness without bulk. Many Water-ruled personalities suffer from a measure of insecurity, so textures and fabrics that impart coziness and a sense of safety may have an enormous healing influence on this type.

Most Water souls are physically responsive to shiatsu or any type of massage utilizing a pressure-point system. They dislike being mauled, pummeled, or rolfed. Light, even strokes over especially cramped areas are beneficial as well. Additionally, reflexology or foot massage that utilizes a system of pressure points is beneficial to subconscious Water types, especially those with prominent Pisces, which rules the feet.

An easy, stress-releasing pressure-point exercise for the Water-ruled personality is as follows:

With your thumbs, find the two hollows on either side of the top of the bridge of your nose. Inhale, hold and press down to a slow count of ten. Release and exhale.

Find the hollows at your temples. Press down to a count of ten, breathing as above and release.

Find the hollows on either side of your nostrils at the base of your cheekbones. Press down to a count of ten and release.

Find the hollows at the base of your earlobes. Press down to a count of ten and release.

Finally, find the hollows on either side of your jawbone about at the midway point, press down to a slow count of ten, breathing as in step one and release.

The Sense of Smell

Aromatherapy is most useful for the Water-ruled personality, since the techniques and practices involving fragrance are non-invasive, gentle, and don't require a lot of extra effort from a personality type whose energies are frequently at a premium. Still, scented oils, worn as perfume, added to the bath (Water types just love baths . . .), simmered in a potpourri, or carried fresh will all do much to stimulate, invigorate, create a sense of calm and security, and serve to center Water's delicate nervous system.

Aromas may be targeted to specific ailments and disorders as charted below, but for general tonic and inhalant purposes, the Water-ruled would do well to surround themselves with the scents of freesia, gardenia, rose, geranium, hyacinth, iris, lily, ginger, lemon, magnolia, myrhh, and ylang-ylang.

All of the above should provide both a calming and centering influence for Water personalities. For the occasional lift in energy level and spirits try essence of orange, vanilla, or white musk.

Consult the suggestions and recipes later in the chapter for further specifics and refer to the Monthly Healing Ritual for Water on page 166.

Aroma Remedies for Specific Water Ailments

AILMENT	ESSENCE	FORM
Back Pain	Neroli, Rosemary, Lavender	Inhalant
Bronchitis	Lemon, Eucalyptus, Clove	Tea infusion
Diarrhea	Thyme, Chamomile, Oregano	Tea infusion
Depression	Basil, Thyme, Marjoram	Fresh or cooked
Lack of energy	Thyme, Orange, Jasmine	Tea infusion
Toxicity	Garlic	Fresh or cooked
Water retention	Chervil, Parsley	Fresh or tea

Recipes for Water Healing

Rose Almond Dates

An excellent remedy for Water-ruled depression, this will reduce the craving for sweets without the use of refined sugars.

1 pound dried dates, pitted
1 pound whole unblanched almonds
Enough rosewater to cover dates, approximately one cup

Make your own rosewater by infusing 8 ounces of rose petals in 1 pint of boiling water for 10 minutes. Strain and pour over the dates. You may use distilled, commercially available rosewater if you prefer. Allow the dates to stand uncovered overnight. Drain and stuff the dates with the blanched almonds. A wonderful source of physical and emotional strength.

Garlic Soup

A time-honored recipe from France, where its health benefits are touted as being competitive with, if not superior to, chicken soup. Especially useful for detoxifying the system, it strengthens the immune system, offering protection against colds, flu, and bronchial ailments.

6 large garlic cloves, peeled and pressed
3 cups water
1 tablespoon tapioca
**½ teaspoon dried thyme, or 1 teaspoon fresh thyme
     leaves**
2 tablespoons sweet butter or virgin olive oil
Black pepper, freshly ground
Parmesan or gruyere cheese, grated, to taste

Place the garlic and the water together in a
saucepan and simmer over low heat for twenty minutes. Add the tapioca and thyme and simmer for an
additional ten minutes. Stir in the butter or olive oil
and top with the ground pepper and cheese. Serve
very hot.

Gem Elixirs for the Water-Ruled Personality

A gem elixir is made by dropping a crystal or stone
of one's choice into distilled water, wine, or brandy
for up to seven hours. This allows the properties of
the stone to be released into the liquid. Many
Water-ruled personalities prefer to take their crystal
energy in liquid, rather than tactile, form, as it is
more in keeping with the natural flow of their energy.
Crystal and gem elixirs are highly volatile and once
made, the bottle should be shaken vigorously to
activate and release the energies within before consuming the elixir.

Diamond, quartz, rose quartz, or preferred gemstone
1 pint distilled water, brandy, or white wine
1 sterile clear-glass container with a glass stopper

Choose a time when the sun or moon is in a Water sign. Cleanse the stone or crystal by dipping in salt and rinsing in clear running water. Drop the stone into the clear-glass bottle, fill with the liquid of your choice and place on a sunny windowsill or under a pyramid for seven hours to release the stone's energy. Gem elixirs should be taken morning, noon, and before bed for at least seven days to be effective.

Baths for Water Healing

Herbal Water Bath

The bath should be an essential part of the Water-ruled personality's healing routine. Three times a week is recommended for Water-ruled personalites; every day is preferred.

Under hot running water add 3 drops of oil of violet, 4 drops of oil of rose, and 1 or 2 drops of oil of jasmine. Add a handful of eucalyptus leaves and a sprinkling of fresh rose petals to the water.

Cleansing Water Bath

Sensitive Water souls should cleanse themselves of other's vibrations with some regularity.

Under running water add 1 handful of pure sea salt, 1 handful of plain baking soda, and 3 drops of oil of violet. Bathe by the light of a white candle inhaling incense of High John the Conqueror for protection and healing. Dry with white towels.

Water Breathing

An excellent short-term stress reliever, this simple exercise can also be used as a prelude to meditation.

> Stand facing forward, arms hanging loosely at your side, knees unlocked. Inhale to a count of six, while raising your arms in an arc until the backs of your hands meet above your head. Do not bend your elbows. While holding your breath, stretch to a count of three, and exhale slowly to a count of nine, concentrating on blowing the air out through your navel. Repeat three times.

Water Affirmations

Simple key phrases, repeated to yourself in meditation or throughout the day, can do a great deal to keep yourself aligned with the natural energy of the Water element. Again, these are only a few examples, use them to build your own personal power phrases.

> *I surrender to the sea of greater consciousness.*
> *I will respond only to positive suggestions and vibrations.*
> *Knowledge and understanding is within me.*
> *Inner harmony is the natural state of my being.*
> *I dissolve with Water's power all feelings of envy, fear, and hate.*
> *I am able to release all tensions and resentments.*
> *I am surrounded by a circle of loving, supportive energy.*

The Fire Personality

PASSION IS WHAT MAKES THE FIRE PERSONALITY TICK. THEY inspire it in others, crave it for themselves, and believe the world would be a far better place if life were played a whole lot more like an opera and a whole lot less like the school pageant.

"You gotta have heart . . . " are the lyrics to the popular song, and Fire personalities have it. Lots of it. Fire rules the third, or heart, chakra. While their emotions may sometimes lack the depth of, say, a Water personality's, or the breadth of their perceptions the natural scope of the Air type's, they never lack for excitement.

Natural leaders, it is the Fire soul's quest to inspire and motivate other people. They are here to take center stage, cheer us up, love us, and get the world off its derriere. They are hugely charismatic, wonderfully brave, and unbelievably optimistic. There is something incredibly resilient about most Fire personalities; these people are capable of an almost phoenix-like comeback from the worst of reverses, losses, and setbacks.

This can be a fortunate trait, since many Fire types burn so brightly and with such intensity that they will almost certainly have to resurrect themselves from their own ashes at some point during their lives. While the Fire personality's dedication, natural fearlessness, and sheer guts makes them truly gifted at getting what they want, they tend to get it at their own expense—*especially* at their own expense. Burning the candle at both ends is a rather mild description of Fire's capacity to exhaust its own energies. Fire often seems to have a secret conviction of its own immortality, a quality that can lead them to a complete disregard for common sense when it comes to getting enough rest, eating right, and avoiding overindulgence. Staying healthy often takes a back seat to living on the edge. Scorning the dubious comforts of a more cautious life-style, the Fire-ruled have a deep and abiding need to feel utterly, completely, and totally alive, which, in actual practice, can leave them depleted, burnt out, and totally exhausted.

Nonetheless, the Fire-ruled personality conceives of itself as self-sufficient and indestructible. They are neither. For it is in the nature of Fire to need fuel and refueling and truer still that without nourishment even the most raging inferno can ultimately be extinguished. Yet curiously enough, Fire has almost no notion of defeat. "Never say die" is Fire's motto, and it is sometimes necessary for cooler heads to bring them to their senses when the war of the moment is lost, the field is strewn with the dead and dying, and everyone else has packed up and gone home.

Fire truly needs others to burn at its brightest. They require and want adulation, appreciation, and the admiration of lesser mortals, though not for purely egotistic reasons. It simply makes them feel better, more complete, and more alive to have armies to lead, forces to garner, and battles to wage. Fire illuminates injustice, after all, and inspires others to action. In fact, the Fire personality believes that any problem can be solved with action—that it is always better to do something, rather than nothing. Watching and waiting are two words not often found in the Fire-ruled personality's vocabulary.

They are impatient, headstrong, and big-hearted. Conversely however, it is their innate self-centeredness that can make them the most selfish of any of the elemental types, though not necessarily on a conscious level. It's just that they generally view themselves as strong and self-reliant; they tend not to perceive their own needs, much less anyone else's.

Fire lives in the moment and loves to the end. The most genuinely loving of any of the elemental types, they will move mountains, hang the moon, or burn their bridges in the name of love and romantic passion. When it comes to the dailiness of taking out the garbage, paying the bills, and meatloaf every Wednesday, however, Fire's flame is apt to sputter rather quickly. Don't look to Fire for good habits, steady ways, and emotional stability; they are far more likely to look for opportunities to put a match to whatever emotional or circumstantial powder keg happens to be lying around, purely for the satisfaction of seeing it blow up. Fire craves excitement—when the drudgeries of day-to-day existence don't provide that excitement, they are perfectly capable of making their own.

Though Fire people have been variously described as blunt or even tactless, it is perhaps more accurate to say that they express themselves with an almost naive simplicity. Usually quite verbal, dishonesty nevertheless is practically unknown to this type. They say exactly what they mean, and presume that others do the same—a quality that can leave them in for some rude awakenings as they encounter more devious or manipulative souls. Fire never lies—it can on occasion, however, be prone to exaggeration. And though Fire can indeed rush in where angels fear to tread, they can never be said to hurt or offend intentionally.

Physically, Fire types are usually vigorous, fueled by their inner intensity. This, in turn, is fueled by copious amounts of sunlight (they are more prone to Seasonal Affect Disorder or SAD than any other element); regular, even strenuous, exercise; and frequent doses of the kind of life experience the rest of us might call adventure. They are frequently subject to high blood pressure, stress-related disorders, sexually transmitted diseases, heartburn, and ulcers. Healing that utilizes crystals, colors, and music are all especially effective, because Fire nearly always has a highly developed artistic sense. Even if they have never had the patience or discipline to become artists themselves, they are always among the first to appreciate it. Healing exercises that speak to their sense of beauty and passion will always help restore the Fire soul's uneasy balance and sense of optimism when they fall prey to the kind of disillusionment brought on by life in a slower, more hesitant world.

The Fire/Water Personality

This personality is characterized by a certain emotional unpredictability. Fire needs passion and Water needs to feel and this combination can result in a person who, in his or her search for intensity, is quite capable of blowing love affairs, arguments, and quibbles over the grocery bill completely out of proportion.

Though this configuration does not have quite the same propensity for self-defeating behaviors as the Water/Fire type, it can display a unique talent for "shooting itself in the foot" or "falling apart in the stretch" just when their goals are within reach. They will fight for things they don't especially want, attempt to rally others around a cause they don't particularly believe in, and play the devil's advocate better and more often than any other type.

Still, the Fire/Water type will almost surely drive others crazier than it drives itself. Because, for all its dramatic talent, the Fire/Water personality has a curious ability to remove itself from the fray before it becomes overly entangled in threatening or damaging situations.

Personable, sensitive, and theatrical, the Fire/Water type makes for gifted actors, performers, and orators. For all of their monumental intensity and their ability to make others feel, constancy is not their strong suit; the instant gratification afforded by the performing arts is well-suited to their restless, changeable natures.

Impulsive and often maddeningly illogical, they are extremely sensitive to what others think of them, and you will find the Fire/Water personality taking to their beds weeping and plotting revenge over a rude remark or unintentional slight.

Yes, they are temperamental, even quite manic. They have a lot of conflict concerning issues of freedom and attachment—aspiration and security. But when suitably inspired, they perform the best of any other type under pressure, displaying inner strength, courage, and dedication. Perhaps they push themselves to extremes knowing at some level that this is where they can really outshine the rest of us.

With some encouragement, however, they can learn to moderate a bit in order that they may better encourage others. And when their great sensitivity is taken out of the realm of the purely personal and into a more universal context, Fire/Water is capable of striking those chords that truly resonate in everyone.

The Fire/Air Personality

Idealistic and positive, this person lives at a level of inspiration and intention that is usually above reproach. By and large, the Fire/Air personality really is holier-than-thou, than me, or anybody else, though they are unlikely to point it out unless it is genuinely in the interest of motivating lesser souls to some great cause or ideal. Fire aspires and motivates, Air fans the flame and fuels it with notions of larger context, broader vision, and universal impact.

Fire/Air can and should make its mark in the world, for this type is more capable than any other of making the world a better place. They have the ability to put their ideas into action and to gain, through experience, a real grasp of the implications of their actions. Unlike other Fire-ruled types, this one is able to "look before they leap" and, perhaps more important, to persuade others to leap right along with them.

Yet emotion in this configuration lacks a certain personal quality. For all of Fire/Air's ability to inspire to larger goals, smaller, more personal involvements tend to make them skittish, and they will often neglect the kind of personal life that could prove a source of even greater strength. Here is where you find priests, monks, and holy men and their female counterparts. Here, also, is where you find the cynics and the perennially disillusioned malcontents.

Marked by a keen sense of humor and certain creativity, this type can fall prey to chronic dilettantism in their rush toward the new, the stimulating, and, above all, the intelligent. But it is a configuration that nevertheless lacks depth, not because they do not have the potential for depth, but because they tend to neglect or avoid those aspects of life that might ground them. The emotionalism of Water is something they find too heavy, the practicality of Earth they might find too tedious, yet these are the very qualities than can—and do—provide universal nourishment.

Thus, Fire/Air will find themselves in an almost chronic state of depletion unless they are careful. Nervous, high strung, and often scattered, they will benefit greatly from the essential nourishment of sensual healing as it can return them and ground them in an appreciation of the simple pleasures, rather than a sense of the perils—of the flesh.

The Fire/Earth Personality

While not possessed of quite the same tenacity as the Earth/Fire combination described on page 69, Fire/Earth is nonetheless marked by a formidable vitality, an enormous capacity for work, and a truly inspired approach to life.

The Fire/Earth personality is often marked by a wonderful, raucous, earthy sense of humor. They are curiously difficult people to fool. Unlike some of their other Fiery counterparts, this particular configuration is capable of a kind of "bottom line" perception of situations and people, along with a very low tolerance for deceit, smoke screens, and plain old BS.

Though they may find themselves pining from time to time for the kind of life that would provide them with fewer worries, more romance, and greater freedom, Fire/Earth in fact has a real talent for tending to the details while rising above the drudgery, for maintaining a sense of inner freedom and uniqueness within the demands of a job or the system, and for attending to the needs of others with dedication, love, and devotion without neglecting themselves.

They are more nurturing than other Fire types and an innate physical confidence and grace makes them great doctors, nurses, and physical therapists. From the purely physical point of view, there is very little that grosses these people out. They are tough, confident, and optimistic, and if they don't neglect the more spiritual and emotional aspects of existence, are apt to go far and live long, productive, and wonderfully healthy lives.

When Fire Energy Is Blocked

Fortunately Fire energy is perhaps the least likely of the four elemental energies to get blocked. Fire temperament may be many things, but repressed isn't usually on the list. These people have a wonderful ability to express themselves in the midst of their many emotional ups and downs, and can find or make plenty of opportunities to do so. Still, if Fire people are not often blocked within themselves, the rest of the world has its own ways of repressing, blocking, or trying to extinguish Fire's passion, inspiration, and fervor.

Below is a list of common ailments and complaints that are usually indicative of blocked or over-accumulated Fire energy.

PHYSICAL

Skin disorders such as rashes, eczema, or hives
Heartburn, dyspepsia, or ulcers
Heart disease
Hardening of the arteries
Palpitations
Fevers
Canker sores
Hiccups

PSYCHOLOGICAL

Tantrums
Depression resulting from repressed anger
Unexplained feelings of rage
Excessive competitiveness
Compulsion to be center of attention
Inappropriate generosity or overspending
Exhibitionism
Insomnia
Dominating or overly controlling behavior
Having a "chip on your shoulder"

Fire and the Five Senses

Fire people are usually very much sensually inclined and aware, yet cannot be said to have an especially long attention span for sensually-based activities or indulgences. In healing, then, it is best to keep exercises short and to the point, and to confine Fire to an increased number of short energy-inducing sessions that will fuel their energy before they lose their concentration.

More than anything else, the Fire-ruled personality requires the energies of sunlight to nourish its inmost nature. Though this type may stay out until all hours partying or appear to take very little notice of (or pleasure in) the natural world, they need regular contact with and doses of the energy of the sun to remain in peak spiritual, emotional, and physical form.

Pity the poor Fire personality trapped in a windowless cubicle eight hours a day, or the Fiery party animal whose poor habits keep them out all night to sleep all day. Fire must learn to store up the sun's energy during the summer months by a regime of sunbathing, swimming, and outdoor activity. In the winter months, they need to manage their energy in such a way that they don't burn themselves out by the middle of November. Tanning parlors and solar light will do much to augment Fire energy during the darker times of the year, however, and their use is to be encouraged in any event for the Fire-ruled personality. Many forms of solar light have recently become available for private use and have been used by the medical establishment in curing everything from psoriasis (a classic Fire ailment, by the way) to leukemia and tumors. No one is quite certain just why light treatment is effective, but it is thought that such light triggers certain positive chemical reactions in the hypothalmus. Solar lights are increasingly available worldwide or through your doctor. Be aware that any such light for personal use should generate at least 3,000 lux (a unit of light measure) at a distance of not less than three feet.

The Sense of Sight

Fire responds primarily to the colors yellow and gold in the home environment and would do well to select almost any shade for offices, workspaces, or rooms—like the kitchen and bedroom—where they will be spending a lot of time. Yellow or gold carpets and rugs are also beneficial, as they will draw and ground Fire's sometimes decidedly ungrounded energy.

Fire personalities are cheered by primary colors generally and excited by visual stimuli that others may consider offbeat or even avant-garde. Depending upon their personal tastes, they might consider the inspired color splashes of a Jackson Pollock or the dynamic blend of naive shape and "hot" colors found in Paul Klee or Joan Miró.

Yellow or gold paper lining for a lampshade will provide comfort and cheer to the Fire household and, of course, the rather obvious advantage of a fireplace to provide warmth, cheer, and a focus for Fire energy certainly wouldn't hurt.

Shades of yellow and gold are usually quite complementary to the true Fire personality's ruddy complexion and should be worn whenever possible. Yet as much as Fire like to make an impression, their tastes in wardrobe tend to run down a rather conservative road, probably due to the fact that they are usually too busy with the cause of the moment to pay much attention to the demands of staying *au courant*.

If you simply feel these colors are not for you, try fashionable accessories such as a yellow or gold belt or chain to anchor your energies; a large gold belt buckle worn at the waist will have amazing healing benefits. Equally, gold jewelry of all kinds is wonderful energy for the Fire personality, most especially a pendant or brooch worn over the heart or allowed to dangle just above the solar plexus.

Fire people love "showy" things and anything large and provocative in the way of personal ornament is bound to please. Fire loves crystals and precious stones of all kinds. Indeed, they might be called the magpies of the element group, loving bright, glittery, shiny things in general. Gold jewelry or ornaments that include diamonds, rubies, or fire opals are perhaps the best choices of all.

The Sense of Sound

Fire rules the third chakra and vibrates to the key of E major. Music of scope and passion are good choices here; symphonic works written in that key and, yes, operas are excellent for Fire energy. Stravinsky's *Firebird*, Schumann's *Arabeske in E Major*, and, for quieter moments, Mozart's *Piano Concerto Number 26* in E major will all have a positive influence on aligning and realigning Fire energy. Some Fire people have professed to a great love of flamenco music and dancing—easy enough to understand—considering the passionate nature of Fire. The exciting classical guitar preludes of Hector Villa-Lobos, No. 1 and No. 4 might be good choices here.

Almost to a man or woman, Fire souls love to sing. They may not be any good at it, but they love it anyway. Perhaps they simply love the sound of their own voices—no matter—even the tin-eared Fire personality does him or herself good to indulge in the occasional burst of from-the-gut song.

Buy a pitch pipe and learn the key of E major. Once you've established the key, let yourself go, intoning everything from *hare-krishna hare-rama* to "Runaround Sue" or the drinking song from *La Traviata*. Indulge yourself—with an audience if possible—it'll do you good.

The Sense of Touch

Tactilely, the Fire-ruled personality is not among the more highly evolved of the elemental types. Therefore, they will respond more readily to more obvious, extreme textures in fabrics and clothing. The rough, invigorating texture of a sun-dried terry cloth bathtowel for example, will prove more stimulating and comforting to them than a dryer-fluffed velour; a rough, natural upholstery weave more interesting than a subtle jacquard or damask. Fire is essentially a masculine element, and many of these types can be quite oblivious to the subtler points of textile and textural environment. To touch the sensibilities of Fire energy, go for more obvious textures here, rough, fuzzy, and natural.

Massage techniques such as rolfing (which concentrates on loosening and encouraging flexibility in the connective tissue) are a wonderful choice for the Fire-ruled personality, as it will give them a sense of workout, while simultaneously relaxing them. Swedish and Russian massage are also good, as they tend to be essentially stimulating.

An excellent exercise in self-massage for the Fire-ruled personality is the heart stroke. It is particularly useful in cases of indigestion or mild heartburn. If there is any serious pain or discomfort during this exercise, stop immediately, as it could be indicative of an ulcer or appendix problem.

Lie on your back, feet together, toes pointing toward the ceiling. With your fingertips, gently probe your mid-section, feeling for any points of discomfort. Gently begin to massage around the affected area, lightly stimulating the skin and surface tissue over the stomach, lungs, and breasts, gradually working in wider and wider circles. Finish with long strokes, always working in the direction of and moving energy toward the heart. Enjoy a few moments of deep breathing before resuming normal activity.

The Sense of Taste

As evidenced in these personalities as a whole, the Fire-ruled tend to vast swings of mood and inclinations in their eating habits, ranging from bouts of epicurean splendor and fits of indulgence that would set a Roman to reach for the Maalox, to predawn junkets on the fast food strip in search of cheese fries and belly burgers.

The precepts of moderation are pretty much unknown to the Fire-ruled personality. They will eat everything or they will eat nothing. They are especially fond of stimulants like caffeine and sugar and will put away amounts of coffee, tea, and soft drinks that would strain the kidneys of the average camel. Additionally, most Fire-ruled personalities are convinced that they require huge amounts of animal proteins in the form of rare red meats or greasy fried chicken, but this is not necessarily so. In many cases what the Fire personality does crave is not protein, but the fat associated with animal protein. The consumption of fat literally slows the body down metabolically, and can have a needed calming effect on Fiery mood swings, though obviously they ought to seek other, healthier sources for gentle sedative effects.

What they do need are extra doses of two essential vitamins—vitamin C, which strengthens and augments the immune and nervous systems, and vitamin D, or, as it is more popularly known, "the sunshine vitamin." Fire loves spicy food, and will benefit enormously from dishes that are rich in garlic, onions, ginger, saffron, cumin, and bay. For a *digestif* that is just chock-full of Fire energy try Goldschlager. A liqueur that is cinnamon based (a good Fire spice), it is also flecked with bits of edible 24-karat gold, the combination of which is sure to chase the blues and fan the inner flame of any self-respecting Fire personality. Alternatively, pernod or yellow Chartruese are fine choices.

Fire personalities can and should seek needed vitamins in the forms of extra citrus fruits and whole or low-fat milk, depending upon their individual weight requirements. Fruit will provide needed vitamin C—especially for smokers—and, not surprisingly, many Fire-ruled personalities are smokers. A extra glass or two of lowfat milk per day or the addition of beans and legumes to the diet will also help to satisfy those ravenous protein cravings. For specific recipes and remedies, see pages 132–135.

The Sense of Smell

Not surprisingly, the most effective form of aroma-therapy for the Fire personality will be found in the form of incense. Fire loves fire, loves smoke, and loves all the little accoutrements that go with incense-burning rituals. The use of scented candles is equally recommended, and perfumes that concentrate on fresh, energizing, and spicy scents are all good choices for keeping the energy of the Fire-ruled personality on a more or less even keel.

Specifically, Fire responds well to the warm scents of the sun, whether in incense, candles, or scented oils. Frankincense, clove, sage, bay, rosemary, and the citruses are all good choices here, as are anise, angelica, cinnamon, pettigrain (or bitter orange), juniper, and nutmeg. Flower scents include hibiscus, crocus (saffron), poppy, and marigold.

Aroma Remedies for Some Common Fire Ailments

AILMENT	ESSENCE	FORM
Insomnia	Anise, Hops, Dill	Tea infusion
Heartburn	Fennel, Licorice	Chewed seeds, tea
Skin rashes	Chamomile, Thyme	Applied infusion
Palpitations	Basil, Sage	Fresh leaves, tea
Flatulence	Anise, Cloves, Nutmeg	Tea infusion
Exhaustion	Lemon, Neroli pettigrain	Bath oil or perfume

Recipes for Fire Healing

Herbal "Tobacco"

For those interested in smoking, this all-natural blend will prove a satisfying, less noxious substitute for tobacco.

8 ounces dried coltsfoot leaves
2 ounces dried eyebright leaves
2 ounces dried buckbean leaves
1 ounce wood betony leaves
1 ounce dried rosemary leaves
⅓ ounce dried thyme leaves
½ ounce dried lavender flowers
½ ounce dried chamomile flowers

Blend the mixture thoroughly and rub it through a coarse sieve. Smoke rolled in papers or a pipe. Store tightly covered in a tin or plastic container in the refrigerator.

Insomnia Tea

Mix 1 part valerian with 2 parts hops. Steep in boiling water, 1 teaspoon for every ¾ cup. Sweeten with buckwheat or clover honey, as desired.

Note: This mixture can be somewhat addictive when taken for long periods of time. Do not use for more than 14 days without interruption.

Fire Incense

The simplest way to use this homemade incense is with a charcoal cube and charcoal-incense burner, available in many speciality and religious shops.

Crush 1 cinnamon stick, 1 whole nutmeg, 2 bay leaves, and 4 allspice berries in a spice grinder or food processor. Add 2 ounces powdered sandalwood and ½ ounce powdered orris root. Add a drop or two of rose or poppy oil, if desired. Sprinkle the powder over burning charcoal.

Fire Herb Wine

An excellent tonic wine, full of Fire energy.

1 gallon water
2 quarts chopped sage leaves
2 quarts chopped rosemary leaves
2 quarts marigold petals
6 pounds chopped golden raisins

Boil the water and pour it over the herbs and raisins. Allow the mixture to stand for seven days at room temperature, stirring 2 or 3 times per day. Strain through fine muslin or cheesecloth. Bottle in sterilized containers and secure clean corks with melted paraffin. Allow to mature six months. Decant into fresh bottles, and use as desired.

Baths for Fire Healing

Fire Energy Bath Salts

5 ounces bicarbonate of soda
5 ounces tartartic acid (Cream of Tartar)
3 ounces powdered orris root
4 drops orange or pettigrain oil (if using distilled
    essential oils, use less)
2 drops frankincense oil
1–2 drops orange blossom oil

Mix the above ingredients together. Store tightly
covered and add by handfuls to the bath for a stimulating refreshment.

Fire Breathing

An excellent lung exercise for any element type, the
technique of Fire breathing concentrates on bringing air
in and out of the solar plexus area. Also called bellows
breathing, it is an excellent prelude to Fire meditations
or as a quick way to relieve accumulated tension.
Caution: The first few tries are bound to make you feel
a bit hyperventilated, but as you become more
experienced with the technique, any feeling of light-
headedness will gradually abate.

Drop the head to the chest. Inhale through the
mouth to a slow count of six; exhale through the
right nostril, placing your finger over the left. Pause
for a count of three. Inhale through the mouth to a

count of three; exhale through the left nostril. Pause. Inhale through the mouth, exhale through the mouth, concentrating on bringing the air into and out of your diaphragm. Gradually increase the pace and depth of your breathing until your rate of inhalations and exhalations is like that of a bellows. Work in groups of six breaths; pause for a count of six and repeat, working up to a total of six repetitions.

Fire Affirmations

Even the optimistic Fire-ruled personality needs to give itself a boost from time to time, and these simple affirmations can provide a much needed pat on the back to an element group that, more than any other, tends to neglect or acknowledge its own deepest needs. Use these phrases as guides only, build on them to create your own personal power vocabulary.

My priorities in life are clear to me.
Everything is possible.
I am the creator of my life.
I operate from a space of love and abundance.
I am a channel for the energy of the universe.
Love is my healer; time is my friend.
I am able to see where to best direct my energy.

The Air Personality

IN THE AIR PERSONALITY, COSMIC ENERGY IS EXPRESSED AND actualized in thoughts, concepts, and patterns of perception. Air is comprised of the duality of creative thought and communication—"in the beginning was the Word"—the idea that precedes material manifestation. Whereas the Fire-ruled personality's quest can be said to be one of willing desire into reality, Air's quest can be said to be one of thinking and communicating. They conceptualize and express their ideas to others, thereby ensuring that their ideas sooner or later become reality.

The notion of communication is truly essential to any discussion of the Air-ruled personality. One of the self-expressive pair of elements, talking is as natural and necessary to these people as breathing. Just as the wind will pick up seeds from the ground, carry them along, and deposit them in another place to grow and flourish, the Air-ruled personality will gather and dispense information, somehow transforming the information along the way. Air-ruled personalities are naturally sophisticated, intelligent, and, above all, interested. These are curious people; they love to learn and the process of personal education is never-ending for them.

Air signs and Air-ruled personalities are frequently reported to be rationally and mentally, rather than emotionally or physically, oriented. While to some extent this is an accurate assessment of Air, it can also be said that they have quite the same emotional, physical, and spiritual needs as anyone else. What they also have, however, is a certain ability to detach themselves from those needs when they feel the necessity for gaining greater perspective, a more informed perception, and a broader vision of the workings of life in the world.

The Air-ruled personality is able, as not all others are able, to observe their own and others' lives in an essentially analytic framework. They understand that even in the worlds of emotion and spirituality there are definite rules of cause and effect, of motion and countermotion, and that to discover the secrets of those laws is to broaden understanding.

This fascination for analysis and theory can indeed make the Air-ruled personality seem a bit cold or offputting to some, because it can seem as though the cares and concerns of rest of the world are no more than so many slides under the microscope of these intellectually powerful people. And while it can certainly be said that many an Air-ruled personality has objectified his or her own experience as a means of avoiding deep emotional commitments or other challenges to their sense of freedom, it is this essential objectivity that colors and imparts to the Air-ruled personality a great sociability, more than a little tolerance, and a never-ending interest and curiosity for all types of people from all walks of life.

Objectivity makes for tolerance, and the Air-ruled type is typically free of prejudice, with the possible exception of what might best be termed as intellectual prejudice. They don't like slowness or stupidity nor will they tolerate it for long. While they may have occasion to suffer fools from time to time, you may rest assured they will not do so gladly. Equally, the Air-ruled personality can be put off by—and even rather easily threatened by—those who refuse to appreciate the validity of their thinking or those who insist that an idea or concept must be tested in the material world before it can be considered worthwhile.

In fact, the usually non-emotional Air-ruled can overreact and grow quite paranoid when their opinions are challenged or their theories ignored. They are not famous for their tenacity as a rule, and the harsher aspects of a materially oriented world can send them running to retreat in any number of ivory towers. By and large, they are capable of quite eccentric behavior and can even turn obsessive and fanatical when Air energy is over-accumulated. The example of the slightly dotty, brilliant, and out-of-touch "absent-minded professor" is an excellent example of Air gone wrong or imbalanced.

Air rules the fourth, or throat, chakra: the seat of self-expression. And express themselves they must. For this reason, Air people make brilliant writers and communicators of all kinds, and are especially gifted in the emerging world of computers and the so-called information superhighway. Freedom of thought and expression are essential for this type, and they bear an inherent disaffection for the limits of the harsher aspects of material reality. They can be prone to ignore the needs of the physical body, turn a deaf ear to the emotional needs of loved ones, and show a terrifying disdain for practical matters.

At their best, the Air-ruled personality is delightfully social, wonderfully well-informed, and genuinely interested in those ideas that would better the world. At their worst, they are capable of spending a great deal more time trying to figure out why they are here than they do in actually being here, actively participating in life on the planet.

Sensual healing can do much to anchor the Air-ruled personality in a benevolent understanding of the material, but any exercises or methods ought to be undertaken with an eye to the underlying meaning and thorough explanation of the concept of behind the exercise or method to be utilized. The Air-ruled can be said to be both the most and the least responsive to various alternative healing procedures and methods, having, on the one hand, a fine grasp of the concepts and precepts behind it that will do much to augment the effectiveness of the methods themselves, and, on the other, a generally poor grounding in physical life as a whole. In short, Air people are likely to enthusiastically embrace, thoroughly research, and properly understand the ways and means of spiritual and alternative healing without ever getting down to trying it for themselves. Therefore,

avoid anything that ties them down to a routine or regimen, is unduly strenuous, or relies too heavily on
material objects, for these are the things that are likely to
fall victim to Air's need for flexibility, freedom, and intellectual stimulation. Failing that, sheer novelty can work
wonders. For example, there is currently available a
shareware computer program called Zenware that offers
the user a variety of exercises in meditation and visualization that might spark the interest level of the typical
Air personality, because of the novelty of its approach.

Remember, Air derives its energy from air—from the
world of the invisible, intangible, and ideological. This
personality type has at times been recorded as being
shallow, due to a certain restlessness inherent in the Air
nature. But it is perhaps more accurate to say that in
their quest for intellectual stimulation they can spend
much of their lives gathering information without giving
themselves the necessary time to properly assimilate it.
From the healing standpoint, it is especially beneficial
for these restless souls to withdraw from the outer and
into the inner world of the senses from time to time,
simply in order to give themselves time to think. A simple change of scene will work miracles on these restless
minds. More than any other type, Air needs to "change
the vibrations" from time to time. Boredom and routine
are anathema to these mentally hungry souls. The
opportunity, even for as little as a few hours, to soak up
new environments, new experiences, and new concepts
is essential to their healing process. Having accomplished that much, engaging in the free play of ideas
and discussion can be more pleasurably healing to this
type than to any other single element group.

The Air/Earth Personality

This makes for an extraordinarily rational configuration, and is generally considered quite benevolent, though perhaps not as ultimately materially productive as when Earth is dominant. Nevertheless, the ideals and concepts of Air are here well-grounded and centered in the material world. This individual will go far as an administrator, manager, or in the legal professions. Law enforcement officers, lawyers, and judges are often to be found in the Air/Earth group as they tend to do very well in the application of ideas and ideals in practical and objective reality.

Here Earth lends Air a greater acquaintance with physical needs and desires, and this type is not quite so likely as some others to forget or neglect the physical form. They are far more likely than other Earth combinations to engage in regular physical exercise and are better equipped to recognize common-sense approaches to eating well and getting enough rest in the interest of maintaining health. As a result, most Air/Earth types are blessed with an extraordinary longevity.

Gifted with a dry sense of humor, the Air/Earth type is able to rise above many of the pitfalls of daily encounters with stress and stressors. They have a curious ability to maintain a certain unassailable personal space, even under the most trying of conditions. Logical and able to grasp the complexities of any number of systems of thought, philosophy, and administration, the intellectual and nurturing capacities in the Air/Earth

combination can produce brilliant psychologists, counselors, and social workers. They can, however, neglect
or entirely subjugate their personal lives to their professional ones and are perhaps the most likely to fall prey
to "workaholic" behavior.

The Air/Fire Personality

Optimism in the extreme can be said to characterize
this variation of the Air type, as here the intellectual
aspirations and ideals of Air nourish and complement
the inspirational and motivational qualities of Fire.
These people are smart. Really smart. This is among the
most persuasive, idealistic, and verbal configurations
possible. They make truly wonderful speechwriters,
talk-show hosts, politicians, and soap-box moralists.
The Air/Fire personality is possessed of a singular sense
of the rightness of his or her convictions and can sway
the multitudes with his or her powers of self-expression.
Fire adds a needed note of emotionalism here that can
quite literally put the causes, ideas, and theories of Air
over the top and into the collective imagination.

Of course, once the speech is made, the Air/Fire personality is going to need some help when it comes to
the actual administration and translation of his or her
ideas into reality. Detail-oriented they are most decidedly not, and woe befall any individual to point out to
these volatile personalities just how impossible their
dreams might be when it comes to getting their projects
off the drawing board. These types have big egos and
have been known to shoot the messenger who chal-

lenges the validity of their rhetoric. Many an unsuspecting soul has come in for a truly awesome tongue-lashing as Air/Fire tries to cover the holes in their own logic and planning. They can always win the debate or argument, not because they're right, but rather because they can talk better, longer, and with more conviction than anybody else.

High-strung and prone to nervous disorders of all types, the Air/Fire personality does well to learn the value of simply shutting up and shutting down from time to time—in order to restore their depleted energies. Air needs to think—to step back and take a deep breath—and reckless Fire very often doesn't give it the opportunity. Grounding in physical pleasure can be crucial for these people. Without it, this combination can quite easily burn out of control.

The Air/Water Personality

Air/Water energies can be quite complementary as here Water helps to personalize the intellectual capacities of Air and Air lends a note of detachment and freedom to Water's need for security.

These people have a wonderful grasp of human nature and are capable of great, informed intuition about personalities and situations. On the whole, however, they cannot be said to have as great a degree of awareness about themselves as they do about others, finding it easier perhaps to conceptualize from a distance the human faults, frailties, and behaviors to which we all are susceptible.

Air/Water will usually indulge in a great many experimental and even downright inappropriate relationships in their lives, believing that we are all here primarily to learn from one another—sometimes to the detriment of their own real emotional needs. Nonetheless, when properly aligned, Air and Water energy can combine in an individual who is idealistic, intuitive, inspirational, and emotional. Like its Water-dominated counterpart, Air/Water can be an impractical dreamer, yet in the Air-dominant configuration one is more likely to find an eccentric rather than a real escapist, or a mere cynic rather than a genuine malcontent.

At best, this type is gifted with an active and productive creative imagination, and may excel in the arts. They make excellent healers and counselors, as their intuition about people can be brilliantly and concisely expressed.

Physically, this type is perhaps the most physically and psychologically sensitive. Attuned on some vital level to all things invisible, they can pay dearly when their equilibrium is upset by poor environment, destructive atmosphere, bad vibrations, or ill will. This is the type who really will sicken and die from a broken heart or a witch doctor's curse. Those two events being relatively rare in most lives, however, they still need the benefits of preventive healing and spiritual protection—on the spiritual, emotional, and physical planes.

When Air Energy Is Blocked

Air energy is characterized by its intellectual prowess and its need to communicate a wealth of information, ideas, and concepts. Over-accumulation of, or blocked Air energy will be indicated by an over-involvement in the affairs of the material world, an inability or lack of desire to express one's thoughts, and most especially by obsession or fixation on a particular idea, person, or concept. Air difficulties may also be indicated a lack of cooperation, preoccupation or chronic dissatisfaction with close personal relationships, and an inability to gain perspective or adjust to change in the form of new ideas, new people, and new ways of doing things in the workplace. Equally, thinking too much or a paralysis of will can be another indication of over-accumulated Air energy.

Below is a list of common complaints and ailments indicated by blocked or over-accumulated Air energy.

PHYSICAL

Asthma
Throat troubles of all kinds
Inability to speak
Laryngitis
Tonsillitis
TMJ
Neck or shoulder pain
Gum disease
Lung and upper bronchial disturbances
Nervous-system disorders

PSYCHOLOGICAL

Inability to cope with change
Attention deficit problems
Obsessions and fixations
Lack of mental discipline
Inability to organize priorities
Over-thinking
Feeling threatened by new concepts or precepts
Overactive imagination or delusions of grandeur
Difficulty with objectivity or gaining perspective
Destructive behaviors brought on by boredom or
    routine
"Shopaholic" behavior

Air and the Five Senses

While the Air-ruled personality may not always be
entirely sure or even remotely conversant with its inner
needs, there is one thing on which you can rely: They
know—and are usually able to tell you in twenty-five
words or less—what they like. And without exception,
one of the things they like is variety. Lots of it. New
faces, places, languages, concepts, and ideas all excite
the Airy mentality and serve to enhance its natural
energies. A new outfit, a new cuisine or restaurant, a
new haircut or makeup, even a new briefcase can help.
In fact, many Air-ruled personalities, while not especially materialistic, love to shop and can be inveterate
shopaholics under the right circumstances. This is not
because they are especially materialistic or especially

trying to augment their needs for security, but simply because they thrive on the new. Newness or novelty empowers and refreshes these souls. In a very real sense, they require change for its own sake. Perhaps it is qualities like this that give rise to notions of Air's shallowness. Yet because things are sometimes done for obvious reasons doesn't make them any less valid.

The Sense of Sight

The need for variety in an Air-ruled personality's life can sometimes express itself in a personal environment that is often terribly cluttered. Active and mentally agile Air types don't often hold neatness or order very high on his or her list of personal priorities, but like to be surrounded with the variety they crave. Decorating schemes, if they exist at all, tend to embrace the eclectic and even the eccentric at one extreme, or find expression in overly conceptualized fashions-of-the-moment that do not always allow for needs or personal comfort. Whatever the individual approach to the specifics of Air-based interior design, they should attempt to incorporate the colors of the fourth chakra at every opportunity.

Cool greens, aqua, and blue-green are excellent choices both in the work or home environment or as part of the individual wardrobe, and will provide a healing influence to the Air type. Green is the color of growth and renewal. It has a tranquilizing effect on the nervous system and beneficial effects upon the circulation. Green is such a beneficial color that it has a wide range of healing uses for almost any element group, but is especially beneficial to the nervous, restless, and sometimes disorganized energies of Air. When at all possible, Air work and personal areas should have a feeling of space—or airiness, as it were. Failing the square footage, however, Air might consider a ceiling or electric fan placed at a strategic point in the home or office, and, yes, keep the windows open—whatever the weather. Equally, Air embraces all highly conceptualized forms of environmental decor and might consider a further study and use of such disciplines as the Oriental art of Feng Shui, which will doubtless appeal to their intellectual, if not their aesthetic, sensibilities. Computer art, animation cells, and abstractions are all especially good choices for the Air-dominant personality, and many respond well to the work of surrealists.

The Sense of Sound

Not many Air types have a highly developed sense of sound or fine musical ear, primarily because they are far better at speaking and expressing themselves than they are at listening. Nonetheless, the Air-ruled can benefit enormously from the vibrational forces of sound and music and are especially responsive to the tonal experiments found in a great many New Age recordings, particularly *Pan Flute* by La Mir or *Fairy Ring* by Mike Rowland.

Novel sounds fascinate this personality group, just as they are fascinated by novelty in other areas. They like percussion and might do well to invest in a rain stick, gourd rattles, or drums for personal meditation exercises.

Air rules the fourth chakra and vibrates to the key of F major. Classical selections for an Air-ruled personality might include many of the works of Scriabin or Debussy, most especially the popular *Claire de Lune*. More traditional Air types might appreciate Mozart's *Piano Concerto* No. 19 in F major or Beethoven's *String Quartet* in F major, Opus 18.

The Sense of Taste

Unlike the other element groups, Air personalities will do well to increase, rather than decrease, the amounts of proteins in their usually haphazard diets. For those concerned about their intake of animal fats, this is best accomplished by incorporating protein in the form of legumes and nuts, though fish, most particularly shellfish, is also to be encouraged.

The Air-ruled personality will also benefit from greens of all kinds, and most especially from the extra iron found in spinach, beet, mustard, and collard greens, as the group shares a tendency to anemia with the Earth-ruled.

Though the Air personality is unlikely to overeat, they may go through times when they forget to eat properly or, indeed, eat at all. Their sensitive metabolic balances are much improved by the intake of several small meals or snacks throughout the course of a day, rather than tying themselves to the routine of two or three larger and heavier sessions at the table.

They love experimenting with new foods and cuisines and you will find the typical Air personality rushing off for anything from tapas to sushi at the first suggestion. They can neglect proper diet, however, when they fall prey to the dubious nutritional value of fast and frozen foods consumed directly from the microwave in a standing position.

Air people, with their fascination for the high-concept approach to anything and everything and their love of the new, can go on odd food fads or embrace the flavor-of-the-month with an enthusiasm that is not always healthy. Weird diets appeal to them; they are often guilty of trying them out of curiosity—just to see if they'll work. The same holds true for the latest rage in health food, vitamins, or Amazonian miracle herbs. Air-ruled personalities believe in miracles, you see, and they're always on the lookout for the latest in discoveries and cure-alls. The simplicity of things like a balanced diet and fresh whole foods is boring by comparison.

Nevertheless, Air people do well to eat lightly and with some regularity. They, more than any other group, ought to avoid stimulants like caffeine that give them an illusion of energy when they are already extended far beyond their normal capacities. Calmative herb teas like chamomile and yerba mate are very beneficial, while disturbed sensitive Air digestion can benefit from a *digestif* like Sambucca or Anisette. Green Chartreuse, both for its color and its base incorporating the Air-ruled herbs of fennel, hyssop, angelica, and lemon verbena, can be considered a superb selection. Further, any of the herbs that are traditionally associated with general tonic properties or longevity are especially appealing and compatible with Air energy. Good choices here include: ginseng, gotu-kola, and, yes, garlic for its benefits to the circulatory system.

The Sense of Touch

Air, like Water, is an element group that can be called almost hypersensitive when it comes to fabrics, materials, and texture. Subtle weaves here; nothing scratchy, coarse, or spongily synthetic will be found acceptable under those super-charged fingertips. Kidskin or lamb-suede, please. Nothing stiff or inflexible. They are especially fond of the unusual, though, and may take an unexpected shine to a pair of ostrich leather cowboy boots or an ottoman upholstered in python bellies. For the basics though, stick to sheer curtains (they adore chiffon), light, unobtrusive textures, and, above all, choose things you don't mind replacing, as Air changes its mind about its personal tastes and preferences the way other people change socks.

Massage-wise, Air responds to pressure-point massage (a short session please, they don't sit still for long) and they will benefit more than any other element group from the use of vibrators or massage beds. They may find specifically sensual massage as an excellent prelude to intercourse as well, as it has the function of "getting them back in their bodies" and making these somewhat less than physical types more comfortable with physical forms of intimacy.

The Sense of Smell

Perhaps the best choice for healing the Air type is aromatherapy. Scent, fragrance, and aroma are comprised of essence and the air itself. They are closest to Air's natural energy and element, and they will have powerful, positive effects on the typical Air-ruled personality.

Therefore, scent in all its forms, oils, essences, inhalants, potpourris, perfumes, and incense will work wonders on a stressed-out, depleted Air soul. Consider the ephemeral healing joys of a pocket full of eucalyptus leaves or a carnation in your buttonhole; the way a sniff of lush lily-of-the-valley can change the inner, if not the outer, landscape of a grey winter's day to a sunny April afternoon. Scent has the further advantage for Air types of being effortlessly incorporated into their lives without the cumbersomeness of, say, a crystal collection or a personal apothecary.

Suggestions for specific treatments of specific ailments are included below, but for general tonic and healing purposes, the Air-ruled personality should surround him or herself with the fresh, neutral aromas of carnation, mint, parsley, celery, lemon balm, lemon verbena, anise, meadowsweet, and eucalyptus. Other choices might include: angelica, licorice, savory, and sweet marjoram.

Aroma Remedies for Common Air Ailments

AILMENT	ESSENCE	FORM
Hoarseness	Horehound	Tea or candied
Sore throat	Celery, Ginger, Lemon	Tea or gargle
Toothaches	Coriander	Chewed leaves
Nervousness	Chamomile, Peppermint	Tea
Poor Circulation	Parsley, Sage	Tea
Bronchitis	Mint, Eucalyptus, Rosemary	Tea
Poor concentration	Sweet marjoram, Meadowsweet	Inhalant

Recipes for Air Healing

Herb and Leek Soup for Air Energy

Purported to have healing qualities for the fourth chakra area, this is used by opera singers before a performance for its powerful benefits to the throat.

1 medium onion
1 small bunch leeks, washed and trimmed
2 garlic cloves, peeled
1 pint goat's milk
2 tablespoons olive oil
1 bunch fresh hyssop, washed and chopped fine

Chop the leeks and onions together in the food processor or by hand; add the garlic cloves. Add them to the warmed goat's milk along with the olive oil and cook just until the vegetables are tender. Add the hyssop and, if desired, a little salt. Serve warm.

Pan-Roasted Fennel

Fennel is excellent for the digestion and for the promotion of muscular energy. This is especially recommended after over-exertion.

2 large fennel bulbs, trimmed and halved
2 cloves garlic, crushed
¼ cup extra-virgin olive oil
Sea salt
Pepper, freshly ground
2 ounces gruyere or parmesan cheese, freshly grated

Boil the fennel bulbs in salted water for 15 minutes. Drain well. Rub the inside of a sauté pan with the garlic, add the olive oil, and heat. Cook the fennel bulbs for an additional 15 minutes over a medium flame until they begin to caramelize, turning often. Sprinkle with the cheese, cover the pan, and turn off the heat. Keep the pan covered just until the cheese melts. Salt and pepper as desired.

Antiseptic Mouthwash

Air-ruled personalities are especially prone to sore throats, halitosis, gingivitis, and diseases of the mouth and gums. This simple-to-make mouthwash will aid in healing all of the above problems and then some.

1 cup distilled water
3 tablespoons white wine vinegar
6 cloves, lightly bruised
1 cinnamon stick
2 teaspoon lemon juice

Make a decoction by boiling the above ingredients together over a low flame for 10 minutes. Cool and store in the refrigerator. Use as a mouthwash or gargle twice a day.

Air Sachet

Combine 2 ounces of lemon verbena with the heads of a half dozen carnations. Add 2 teaspoons of dried sweet marjoram. Add 2 drops of anise oil. Mix and place into sachet bags.

Baths for Air Healing

Energizing Air Bath

Under running water, add two drops of peppermint oil or extract, a drop or two of lemon or rosemary oil, and a handful of eucalyptus leaves. An additional drop of rose geranium oil may be added if desired.

Calming Air Bath

Under running water, add 3 drops of meadowsweet oil, 2 drops of chamomile oil, and 1 drop of lily-of-the-valley oil. Sprinkle the surface of the water and add a handful of lemongrass or rose petals.

Air Breathing

The Air-ruled personality doesn't usually require too much in the way of breathing exercises or instructions, but can benefit from the use of the following exercise as a prelude to relaxation or meditation.

Sit in a quiet place in a comfortable position. Allow yourself to become fully aware of your breathing, listen to it, feel it, allow its energy to course through you. Inhale to a count of eight, concentrating on inhaling green glowing light. Hold the breath and exhale, pursing your lips and forcing the air from your lungs in a series of eight short puffs while concentrating on exhaling dark or negative energy. Repeat four times.

Air Affirmations

Though often not highly aware of its own needs, the Air-ruled personality benefits enormously from verbal reassurances found in the use of affirmations; they will derive healing energy from the occasional conversation with themselves. Use the list below to build and create your own affirmation vocabulary.

I am healthy, wise, and loving of myself and others.

I have a body; I am more than a body.
I have a mind; I am more than a mind.
I have emotions; I am more than emotions.

All that I need, I draw to me.
All that I have, I give away.
All that I give, comes back to me tenfold.

All is one and I am one with all that is.

Each breath I take brings me nearer to awareness and understanding.

The Monthly Healing Rituals

YOU HAVE PROBABLY ALREADY DETERMINED THAT THE REAL value of sensual healing is as preventive medicine. After familiarizing yourself with the foregoing chapters, I hope you will agree that regular, moderated sensory indulgence will provide a non-invasive, pleasurable daily antidote to the subtly erosive and debilitating effects of stress, sensory assault, and the ordinary, day-to-day pressures of modern living.

Above all, know that the process of nourishing your natural energy field should be a constant priority in your life. The art of being simply good to yourself—buying yourself flowers, surrounding yourself with wonderful scents, wearing a color that pleases you, or hanging a favorite picture on a wall—can all serve to augment and fortify the body, mind, and spirit. All of those things do heal, and can help you be more completely who you are in the universe.

Therefore, I hesitate to put forth anything so complicated as a "ritual." The exercises and suggestions contained in this chapter are not rituals in the sense that they are religious, complicated, or invasive. Rather they are (or ought to become) rituals in the sense that they can be incorporated into your regular schedules and easily worked into your personal routines. I hope these healing activities will become as important a part of your attention to your personal health and well-being as going to the gym or getting regular check-ups at the dentist or doctor.

I recommend you set aside time to complete the full ritual or routine for your element or element combination at least once a month, though, of course, you ought to feel free to indulge yourself more often should you feel the need.

The monthly healing ritual is time that you set aside for yourself—to be with yourself. It should be quality time, where you withdraw from your ordinary activities and obligations simply for the purposes of enjoying your own company—of pampering and giving yourself pleasure, getting in tune with and aligning your personal energy to the point where it vibrates more completely with Universal Energy—The Life Force.

The Healing Ritual for Earth

WHAT YOU WILL NEED

Red flowers
Olive oil
Sea salt
Baking soda
Oils of lilac, cinnamon, mimosa, nutmeg, or sandal-
    wood
Cosmetic mud or clay mask using aloe, apricot,
    or chamomile (see recipe below or purchased).
Pure castile or olive oil soap
Personal crystals or jewelry, especially garnet or
    ruby
A comfortable robe or wrap

Clay Mask

Powdered green cosmetic clay is readily available
from pharmacies and specialty shops. Mix with
enough purified water to make a paste. Add ½
ounce aloe vera gel and two drops of the essential
oil of your choice.

The Ritual

Choose a time when either the sun or moon is in one of
the Earth signs—Taurus, Virgo, or Capricorn. Allow
yourself at least one hour of uninterrupted time when
you can be completely alone, or with a significant other
of similar energy.

The day that you plan to do your healing ritual, buy red flowers on your way home. Arrange them attractively in a vase and keep them near you.

Begin by drinking two eight-ounce glasses of water. Allow yourself a few minutes of gentle stretching, toe touches, side-to-sides, deep knee bends, etc. You needn't get strenuous; simply concentrate on those areas of accumulated tension and on increasing your flexibility.

Follow with a glass of ruby port or red wine if you wish. Sit in the middle of the floor and simply relax for a few minutes to a favorite recording, preferably one written in the key of C major. Concentrate on the music; hum along and bring the sound up from the base of the pelvis through the top of the skull. Continue to surround yourself with music during the entire ritual.

When you feel ready, light a red candle. Warm ½ cup olive oil to a comfortable temperature on the stove or in the microwave. It should feel quite warm, but not hot on the inside of your wrist.

Take your candle with you and extinguish any electric lights. Remove your clothing and stand in front of a mirror. If it makes you uncomfortable seeing yourself entirely naked, begin by using a mirror that reflects only your head and shoulders. Stand on a clean white or red towel. Begin by pouring a few tablespoons of the warmed oil on the crown of your head. Massage the oil over your scalp in a clockwise circular motion. Continue pouring the oil over your head, massaging in circles until your skin is completely covered, navel, feet, toes, armpits, everything. Feel the warmth of the oil against your skin. Enjoy the pleasure of its comforting, slippery feel. Look at yourself in the mirror, shining with oil. Smile.

Apply the cosmetic clay mask to your face and as much of your body and hair as you wish. Avoid the eye area. Feel the coolness of the mud tightening your pores and cleansing your skin of impurities. Look at yourself, covered with mud, the earth creature by candlelight. Smile. Laugh if you want to. After all, you are in your element.

Raise your arms high above your head and stretch, inhaling deeply as you do so. Bring your arms back down slowly, feeling the tension drawn out of your body through your pores and into the hardening clay.

When you feel it is time to rinse off the oil and clay, run a hot bath adding equal amounts of sea salt and baking soda. Add 4–5 drops of any combination of earth oils recommended above. Choose a flower or two from your bouquet and scatter the petals over the surface of the water.

Submerge yourself in the tub, head and all. Come up for air and feel your energy level rising to the surface of the water as you do so. Soak for a few minutes, holding a crystal or stone in your left hand. Place the stone in your navel for a few minutes if you desire. Focus on the stone and feel its energy coursing through you.

Silently repeat your personal earth affirmations, or say them aloud if you are with someone else. Begin to wash yourself, or if you have a partner, wash each other with the soap. Visualize any negativity, stress, or anxiety rinsing away in the dissolving clay, condensing in the oil floating on the surface of the water. Rub the flower petals against the surface of your cleaned skin.

When you are ready, stand up and wrap yourself in a red or white towel or a favorite robe. Drain the tub and watch the oily, dirty water disappear down the drain, taking your cares and negative energy with it. You are feeling relaxed, energized, and whole.

Apply the earth oil of your choice to your pulse points—wrists, neck, and temples. Trace a circle of oil around your navel and feel yourself drawing in powerful, positive energies from that point.

Taking your candle and music along, go to another room where you can lie down comfortably on the floor. A massage would be appropriate here if you are working with a partner. If not, take a few moments for self-massage.

Practice the Earth breathing exercise on page 88. Place your hands lightly just below your navel, feeling the air as it pushes in and out. With your hands or with a crystal, push your energy upward toward your navel, your solar plexus, your heart, and your throat. Feel the energy flow from point to point. (It may take some practice, but with time you will be able to sense the flow of energy from chakra to chakra.)

As you feel the energy flow through you, take a few moments to savor the awareness of your senses. The touch of the fabric against your skin, the coolness of the air, the glow of the candlelight, the sound of the music. Experience yourself fully in this heightened state of sensory awareness.

Take a final few minutes to meditate. Relaxed, utterly secure and aware, open your mind to any thoughts, feelings, or impulses that come to your consciousness. Remember them and record them if you wish.

Before retiring or continuing with your activities, have a cup of tea made from a decoction of cinnamon, nutmeg, orange peel, and chamomile flowers.

For Earth/Air Healing

Substitute eucalyptus oil for one of the essential oils above. To the cleansing bath add two drops of green food coloring, or use green tinted soap. In addition to the flower petals, scatter a handful of fresh mint leaves in the water. Incorporate a bloodstone or malachite to use with the garnet or ruby. The healing tea should be made from the above ingredients, eliminating the orange peel and using mint or lemongrass as the base.

For Earth/Water Healing

Always use red roses in the healing ritual described above. Substitute oil of jasmine for the cinnamon oil in the bath and change the ratio of sea salt to baking to one quarter sea salt to three quarters baking soda to raise the alkaline levels in the water. Depending upon the ratio of earth to water in the chart, an oatmeal or cucumber mask can be substituted for the clay, and orange candles (instead of red) would be beneficial.

For Earth/Fire Healing

Eliminate the two glasses of water prior to beginning the healing ritual. Use red carnations for the healing flower. Orange oil should be added to the bath water and a handful of basil leaves should be scattered on the water in combination with the flower petals. Clear quartz crystal or rose quartz should be used in addition to garnet or ruby, and it is recommended that two cups of tea be consumed, substituting clove for the nutmeg and rosemary for the chamomile base.

The Healing Ritual for Water

WHAT YOU WILL NEED

Diuretic Infusion (see below)

Orange-colored flowers or mock orange or apple blossoms

An orange candle

Two or three oranges

Sesame oil (Note: If you have a nut allergy, use olive or vegetable oil as a substitute.)

Baking soda

Orange-scented bubble bath (optional)

Gem Elixir of your choice (see page 112)

A loofah or sloughing sponge

Oils of jasmine, gardenia, vanilla, ylang-ylang, or geranium

A piece of fresh ginger

A satin or silk robe or wrap

A white or orange towel

A reflexology chart

Tea made with jasmine, chamomile, and orange peel

Diuretic Infusion

Boil ¾ ounce of fresh leaf lettuce with ½ ounce fresh chevril in a pint of water for 3 minutes. Allow to cool, strain, and serve warm.

The Ritual

Choose a time when the sun or moon is in a Water sign, such as Cancer, Scorpio, or Pisces. Since most Water-ruled personalities are extremely sensitive to the phases of the moon, this healing ritual is best performed on or near the full moon. Perform these exercises alone or with a partner of compatible or similar energy.

On the day that you plan to perform your ritual, buy your flowers. Arrange them attractively and keep them near you.

Begin your ritual by consuming two cups of prepared Diuretic Infusion (see above).

Relax for a few minutes to a favorite recording. Ocean sounds are particularly effective. Lie down, close your eyes, and listen to the sounds of the waves. Feel the water washing over you—feel the tension sliding out of your body as the waves recede.

When you are ready, eat one or two oranges, section by section. Inhale the scent of the orange as you peel them, rub any residual oil on your pulse points—wrists, temples, and neck. Taste the sweetness of the oranges on your tongue, meditate on the notion that you are consuming the sweetness of life itself.

When you feel ready, light your orange candle. Focus your energy upon the flame, and experience its warm glow spreading through your body. Take in the orange energy through your eyes and bring it to your navel. Visualize an orange glow emanating from your navel.

Warm ½ cup sesame oil to a comfortable temperature on the stove or in the microwave. It should feel quite warm, but not hot, on the inside of your wrist.

Take your candle with you and extinguish any electric lights. Remove your clothing and stand in front of a mirror. If it makes you uncomfortable seeing yourself entirely naked, begin by using a mirror that reflects only your head and shoulders. Stand on a clean white or orange towel. Begin by pouring a few tablespoons of the warmed oil on the crown of your head. Massage the oil over your scalp in a clockwise circular motion. Continue pouring the oil over your head, massaging in circles until your skin is completely covered. Feel the heat of the oil against your skin. Enjoy the pleasure of its comforting, slippery feel. Look at yourself in the mirror, shining with oil. Smile.

Now, pour tepid-to-cool water over your head, or stand under the shower if you prefer. Rinse the oil from your skin, concentrating on washing away the accumulated tension and stress. Repeat the warm-oil, cool-water exercise as desired.

Note: You can follow up the warm sesame oil massage with a cool beer shampoo if you like. The Water-ruled personality is especially responsive to the hops in beer; the tingling of the carbonation is very pleasurable and good for the circulation, and it's great for your hair!

Run a hot bath adding a few handfuls of baking soda. Add 4–5 drops of any combination of water oils recommended above. Choose a flower or two from your bouquet and scatter the petals over the surface of the water.

Submerge yourself in the tub, head and all. Come up for air and feel your energy level rising to the surface of the water as you do so. Soak for a few minutes.

With your mind clear and prepared, take two table-spoonsful of the Gem Elixir of your choice. Relax again in the water, feeling the elixir's energy coursing through your veins. Inhale the scent of the flowers, the water. Hold that energy within you. Exhale slowly, feeling your cares, stresses, and negative emotions going out of you, rising and evaporating like steam.

Rub yourself down with the loofah or sloughing sponge, or have a partner do it, gently stimulating the skin and circulation. Feel yourself shedding old cells, old accumulated energy. Imagine that energy dissolving in the healing waters around you.

When you are ready, stand up and wrap yourself in an orange or white towel or a favorite satin or silk robe. Drain the tub and watch the oily, dirty water disappear down the drain, taking your negative energy with it. Mentally say goodbye to those outworn emotions. You are feeling relaxed, energized, and whole.

Apply the water oil of your choice to your pulse points—wrists, neck, and temples. Trace a circle of oil over your diaphragm and feel yourself drawing in powerful positive energies from that point.

Taking your candle and music along, go to another room where you can lie down comfortably on the floor. A massage would be appropriate here if you are working with a partner. If not, take a few moments for self-massage. Work especially on your feet, using a reflexology chart. Rub additional scented oil into your feet and ankles.

Lie down with your eyes closed. Practice the Water-breathing exercises described on page 114. When you are fully relaxed and your mind is clear, call up the mental image or images of anything or anyone that rises from the waters of your subconscious. Visualize that person or situation, allowing the image to expand fully and in detail. Note the particulars of any aspect of the image that you may have failed to notice before. Then imagine a column or stream of orange light connecting your solar plexus with the person or image you have before you. Imagine the light growing bright and stronger with each inhaled breath. See the light changing, flaring up to a brilliant, cleansing, pure white. Then, finally, see the light grow dim, flicker, and die as your unwanted emotional connections are cleared.

Repeat your personal affirmations to yourself or a partner. Working from an area just above your navel, imagine pure orange light moving up through the heart and throat, down to the pelvis. Concentrate on establishing a clear, unobstructed flow of energy through your chakra points. Feel the energy coursing through you and out through your hands and the soles of your feet.

As you feel the energy flow through you, take a few moments to savor the awareness of your senses. The touch of the fabric against your skin, the coolness of the air, the glow of the candlelight, the sound of the music. Experience yourself fully in this heightened state of sensory awareness.

Take a final few minutes to meditate. Relaxed, utterly secure, and aware, open your mind to any thoughts, feelings, or impulses that come to your consciousness. Remember them and record them if you wish.

Complete your healing session with a cup or two of jasmine, chamomile, and orange tea, sweetened with honey. And do treat yourself to the Almond Rose Dates on page 111.

Water/Air Healing

Substitute a drop or two of oil of eucalyptus or mint for one of the flower scents. Use bubble or foaming bath if at all possible, since the foam helps to disperse the oils in the water. Since many Water/Air types are subject to dry and aging skin, use a facial mask of 2 ounces of clover honey blended with 8 drops of jasmine, gardenia, or violet oil. Apply to face and neck with a spatula or with your fingers; allow to dry for a few minutes or until tacky and pat gently, to stimulate the circulation and tone. Rinse well and follow your bath with a moisturizing rubdown of scented sesame, olive, or mineral oil.

Water/Earth Healing

Water/Earth personalities should precede the healing bath with a full run of stretching exercises, preferably yoga. For those unfamiliar with Yoga, I especially recommend the method in the videotape "YOGA: The Art of Living" Vol. I, narrated by Renee Taylor, and readily available at most video rental outlets. Those suffering from the joint pain or circulation problems common to the Water/Earth personality should add 2–3 drops of black pepper or pimento essential oil to the sesame oil and concentrate on the affected area, avoiding eyes, lips, and genitalia.

Water/Fire Healing

Eliminate the diuretic tea. Instead, have a glass of lemonade or orange juice or a small glass of yellow Chartruese. Accompany your bath with the Fire Incense on page 133. Substitute ¼ cup sea salt for an equal amount of baking soda in the bath and use geranium rather than jasmine oil in the bath. Instead of jasmine tea, prepare a mixture of chamomile, cinnamon, orange, and lemon.

Healing Ritual for Fire

WHAT YOU WILL NEED

Yellow flowers (especially yarrow)
A yellow candle
Coconut oil
Pure olive or coconut oil soap
Oils of rosemary, hyssop, marigold, lemon, or peony
Incense burner and charcoals
Fire Incense (see page 133)
Crystal of your choice
Fire Tea (see below)

Fire Tea

2 cups boiling water
½ cup fresh mint leaves
¼ cup spearmint leaves
⅛ teaspoon saffron threads

Infuse the leaves and saffron in the boiling water for five minutes, strain, and drink.

The Ritual

Choose a time when the sun or moon is in a Fire sign, such as Aries, Leo, or Sagittarius. For the Fire-ruled personality it is best if the ritual is performed on a bright, sunny day around noon. If that doesn't fit in with your schedule, light a fire in the fireplace if you have one. These exercises can be performed alone or with a partner of compatible energy.

If at all possible, try to precede you healing ritual with a meal of the Garlic Soup specified on page 111, especially if you are experiencing any problems with indigestion, heartburn, or constipation.

Arrange your flowers attractively and keep them near you. Begin by relaxing for a few minutes to a favorite recording, especially one written in the key of E major. Sing along if you wish, allowing the music within you to flow up from your solar plexus. If you have to play a musical instrument, play a selection in that key. Improvise on the melody if you want.

When you feel ready, light your yellow candle. Focus your energy upon the flame, and experience the warm glow of it spreading through your body. Take in the warm golden energy through your eyes and draw it to your diaphragm and up around your heart. Visualize a golden glow emanating from your heart, feel your heart growing stronger with the energy you are taking in, then project that energy out into the room. Experience yourself as a channel for golden light.

Warm ½ cup coconut oil to a comfortable temperature on the stove or in the microwave. It should feel quite warm, but not hot, on the inside or your wrist.

Take your candle with you into the bathroom or another comfortable location. Remove your clothing and stand in front of a mirror. If it makes you uncomfortable seeing yourself entirely naked, begin by using a mirror that reflects only your head and shoulders. Stand on a clean white or yellow towel. Begin by pouring a few tablespoons of the warmed oil on the crown of your head. Massage the oil over your scalp in a clockwise circular motion, concentrating on the area behind the ears and in the center of the forehead. Continue pouring the oil over your head, massaging in circles until your skin is completely covered. Feel the pleasant heat of the oil against your skin. Enjoy the pleasure of its comforting feel. Look at yourself in the mirror, shining with oil. Smile.

While you are covered in oil, perform some vigorous stretching exercises. A simple aerobic warm-up would be a great choice here. Be careful about slipping on oiled feet, and don't overdo it. Just warm yourself up to the point when your heart rate and respiration are elevated to a pleasant stimulated state. Proceed to your bathroom or steam room if you're fortunate enough to have one, and turn on a hot shower or steam equipment. Allow the room to really become saturated with steam. Sit or stand during your brief steam session, practicing the Fire-breathing techniques outlined on page 134.

When you feel your pores are fully opened and you are fully relaxed, turn off the shower and run a lukewarm bath. Add 5 or 6 drops of the essential oils of your choice. Sprinkle the water with fresh mint leaves or some yarrow blossoms if you have them. Light the Fire Incense. (It's best, by the way, if you keep your incense-burning accoutrements outside the bath while you're steaming).

Soak for a few minutes, until you feel your body temperature return to normal. Wash with the coconut or olive-oil soap, but take care not to be overzealous in scrubbing. Leave a thin imperceptible film of oil on your body as protection against negative energies.

When you are ready, stand up and wrap yourself in a yellow or white towel or a favorite terry cloth robe. Drain the tub and watch the oily, dirty water disappear down the drain, taking your anger, frustration, and negative energy with it. You are feeling renewed, energized, and whole.

Apply the Fire oil of your choice to your pulse points—wrists, neck, and temples. Trace a circle of oil over your heart and feel yourself drawing in powerful, positive energies from that point.

Lie down with your eyes closed. Place the crystal of your choice over your heart center. Practice the Fire-breathing exercises described on page 134, or if you don't feel ready for it, try some simple deep-breathing exhaling with the "auumm" sound until feel your vibrational level increasing. Feel the energy pouring into you from the crystal and relish it. If you are working with a partner, massage is excellent at this point. If not, try some self-massage, working in circles up toward your heart. Concentrate on making yourself ready to receive love—from the universe, from your friends and family, from a specific individual. Remind yourself that you need love, that you want it, that you are deserving of love. Stand in a sunny window if you have one or near the fireplace; imagine golden light pouring out from your heart center and drawing the love you need back to you. See the light flaring up to a brilliant, cleansing, pure white.

Repeat your personal affirmations to yourself or a partner. Working from an area just above your pelvis, imagine pure energy moving up through the heart and throat, and back down to the pelvis. Concentrate on establishing a clear, unobstructed flow of energy through your chakra points. Feel the energy coursing through you, and out through your hands and the soles of your feet.

As you feel the energy flow through you, take a few moments to savor the awareness of your senses. The touch of the fabric against your skin, the coolness of the air, the glow of the candlelight, the sound of the music. Experience yourself fully in this heightened state of sensory awareness.

Take a final few minutes to meditate. Relaxed, utterly secure, and aware, open your mind to any thoughts, feelings, or impulses that come to your consciousness. Remember them and record them if you wish.

Complete your healing session with a cup or two of tea made with mint, spearmint, and saffron, sweetened with honey. Chew some mint leaves or fennel seeds or bulbs as an accompaniment.

Fire/Earth Healing

Add a few broken cinnamon sticks to your bath water and a scant handful of sea or bath salts. Substitute a bouquet of red and yellow carnations for the yarrow flowers and add carnation oil to the bath. Include lemon juice and fennel seeds in the tea.

Fire/Water Healing

Add 3 drops of gardenia or violet oil to the healing bath. Include the visualization exercise for letting go of unwanted emotional bonds (especially anger) as specified for Water, which appears as the first exercise on page 64. Substitute a prepared Gem Elixir for the Fire Incense.

Fire/Air Healing

Include some eucalyptus leaves and baby's breath with your flower arrangement. Use olive oil in place of the coconut oil for the massage portion of the ritual, and alternate aerobic warm-ups with gentler yoga stretches. Consider a computer-aided visual relaxation exercise for meditation, and include lemon and fresh mint leaves in the tea.

The Healing Ritual for Air

WHAT YOU WILL NEED

A flower arrangement including green eucalyptus,
   ferns, and baby's breath or greenery, such as
   princess pine or juniper, depending upon the
   season

A green candle

Pure castile soap

Light mineral oil, such as baby oil
   (see Note below)

Oils of violet, heliotrope, sweet pea, rose geranium,
   and rosemary

A Facial Mask (see below)

A white or green towel

Fresh mint leaves

A vibrator or computer-aided relaxation program
   (optional)

Tea made from a decoction of anise, clove, and
   ginger

Facial Mask

Combine 1 ground cucumber, 2 drops of almond oil,
and some ground fresh mint leaves in a food processor
or blender. Chill lightly before use.

Note for Air Types: Some Air types, despite their
tendency to dry skin, find a full oil massage too heavy
and distasteful. If this is true for you, experiment with

a mister or atomizer using a combination of a light mineral oil (like baby oil) and warm to hot water for the massage portion of this ritual.

The Ritual

Choose a time when the sun or moon is in one of the Air signs—Gemini, Libra, or Aquarius. The Air-ruled personality might prefer to perform their ritual in the early morning or predawn hours, but it is not essential to its success. If you do perform the ritual during daylight hours, consider hanging a green gel or filter over a sunny window to infuse the room with green light. These exercises can be performed alone or with a partner of compatible energy.

Arrange your flowers attractively and keep them near you. Begin by relaxing for a few minutes to a favorite recording especially one written in the key of D major, especially the works of Mozart or Bach. Hum or sing along if you wish, allowing the music within you to come up from your chest, opening up your throat, and flowing out through the top of your head. Place one hand on the top of your head until you can feel the vibration of the tone. Improvise on the melody if you want.

When you feel ready, light your green candle. Focus your energy upon the flame and experience the cool healing light as it spreads through your body. Take in the vigorous energy through your eyes and draw it into your lungs and chest. Visualize a cool green glow radiating through your chest, down to your solar plexus and pelvis, then bring the energy up back through your chakra points and out through the top of your head. Feel yourself growing more centered, more connected, with each breath. Experience yourself as a channel for healing green light.

When you are ready, take your candle with you into the bathroom or another comfortable location. Remove your clothing and stand in front of a mirror. If you have a green gel over a light or window, stand under it for a few minutes, concentrating the light on your chest and upper bronchia, then proceed to the mirror. If it makes you uncomfortable seeing yourself entirely naked, begin by using a mirror that reflects only your head and shoulders. Stand on a clean white or green towel. Begin by pouring a few tablespoons of the warmed mineral oil on the crown of your head. Massage the oil over your scalp in a clockwise circular motion, concentrating on the area behind the ears and in the center of the forehead. Pour or if you prefer, spritz yourself with and oil/water mixture, massaging in circles until your skin is completely covered. Feel the pleasant warmth of the oil against your skin. Enjoy the pleasure of it against your skin. Look at yourself in the mirror, glowing with a light sheen of oil. Smile.

Perform some gentle stretching exercises, concentrating on working the tension from your throat, neck, and shoulders. With your arms extended, make circles with your shoulders, backward and forward, until you feel the tingling that signals a release of tension. Shake out the tension from your limbs, one by one. Be aware of your respiration and take a few additional moments to practice bringing the air deep into your lungs and diaphragm, expanding your breathing capacity.

Apply the facial mask to your face, neck, and chest. Feel its green cool energy entering your pores. Continue to concentrate on your breathing as you prepare your healing bath.

Add 5–6 drops of any combination of the Air oils to hot running water. You may also add some additional mineral oil to the bath, or bubble bath, if you prefer. Keep the vials of oil near you, and as you bathe by the light of your green candle, lift each of the vials to your nose and inhale deeply, concentrating on taking their unique energies deep within you.

When you are ready, stand up and wrap yourself in a green or white towel or a favorite robe. Drain the tub and watch the oily, soiled water disappear down the drain, taking your anger, frustration and negative energy with it. You are feeling centered, energized, and whole.

Apply the Air oil of your choice to your pulse points, wrists, throat and temples. Trace a line of oil up from your chest to your chin and feel yourself drawing in powerful, positive energies from that point.

Lie down with your eyes closed. Place the crystal of your choice over your throat center. A favorite necklace is an excellent choice here. Emerald would be the obvious choice, but since not every Air personality happens to own the Empress Josephine's treasures, substitute any attractive necklace of stone, preferably a green stone set in silver or platinum. Practice the Air-breathing exercises described on page 157, or simply concentrate on some deep breathing, exhaling with the "auumm" sound until feel your vibrational level rise. Feel the energy pouring into you from the crystal or stone and relish it. Feel yourself grounded and enhanced by that energy. Meditate upon the image lying comfortably on a carpet of soft green grass. Feel the pleasant warm breezes stirring the air over your body; listen to its song. Pull the sweet green energy of the grass and the power of the earth beneath it up into body through your spine. Sense the green energy moving through you like sap through a young, graceful, green tree.

If you are working with a partner, massage is excellent at this point. If not, try some self-massage. Most Air types, especially those with a prominent Uranian or Aquarian configuration in the natal chart, will benefit greatly from the electric energies of a vibrator.

Equally, some Air-ruled personalities might choose to perform some part of their meditations in front of a favorite screen-saver or computer-aided relaxation software program. Set the screen colors to a selection of gentle greens and blues, and simply allow your mind to drift, evolving your consciousness as images drift and evolve before you. Record any insights, impressions, or new ideas that come to you during these valuable creative moments. Resolve to communicate these new ideas to others—through speech or the written word.

Follow your ritual with a warming cup of healing tea. Feel the spice warming your throat, chest, and solar plexus, centering and energizing you.

Air/Earth Healing

Add a red rose to your healing bouquet and sprinkle the petals over the surface of your healing bath. To the bath, add a handful of sea salts or pure bath salts. Precede or follow the healing ritual with a salad made with a profusion of leafy greens, especially chicory.

Air/Fire Healing

Prior to the healing bath, include a steam session as specified on page 134. Precede and follow the ritual with two full glasses of water. Substitute some lavender oil for one of the oils above, or sprinkle the bath water liberally with fresh lavender. Add cinnamon or chamomile to the healing tea.

Air/Water Healing

Include a number of favorite flowers in the bouquet, especially lilac, rose, or peony. Omit any bath salt and add a scant ½ cup of baking soda to the bath water. Preceding the ritual with a sauna or steam is excellent. Substitute peony oil for the sweet-pea oil in the bath, and use olive oil in the spritz or massage.

Healing Your Relationships

WE'VE ALL FOUND OURSELVES IN SITUATIONS WHERE we were literally "out of our element" spiritually, physically, and emotionally. The Fiery child growing up with Earth parents; the Airy idealistic employee trying on a daily basis to discern the motives of a Watery emotional supervisor. And of course, the ever-present tendency of opposites to attract in friendships, marriage, and sexual relationships—to feel that we attract those who are "wrong" for us.

Yet from the point of view of elemental energy it may be helpful to realize that just because we find ourselves in situations or relationships that are different or at odds with the way we are used to doing things, it doesn't mean they have to be necessarily bad or have a debilitating effect. In fact, the sensitive Water personality who finds him- or herself involved with Fire-ruled temperaments again and again is not necessarily doing themselves a psychological or emotional disservice. What is far more likely is that they are attracted to Fire energy because they feel the need for that energy in their lives on a very fundamental level.

A practical hard-headed Earth boss may dampen the imagination and creativity of an Air-ruled personality, but in fact that boss can serve a real function in your life if you recognize that his rules and regulations are keeping you in touch with material reality and responsibility. That Fiery lover may exhaust you, but keep you moving, involved, and inspired.

Of course, all such theorizing tends to work better on paper than it does in real life. Long-term intimate relationships tend to fall apart under the stress of constant incompatibility of energy, and that boss can make you neurotic to the point of illness if you let him.

So if you find yourself in a situation where you are constantly exposed to incompatible energies and feel that it is beginning to affect your well-being, try the few simple suggestions below to augment and nourish your personal energy field without putting it at risk for undue conflict.

First and most important, try to obtain the chart or charts of the individual(s) who most concern you. Don't look for incompatible elements, but for common ground. Air/Water employees for example, will find their working life much improved with an Earth/Water boss if they stop trying to analyze or intellectualize what he or she does and recognize instead that sensitivity and more emotional responses (even to professional situations) is perhaps the path of least resistance. After all, these two have Water as a common energy. If they nourish the Watery elements of their relationship, rather than ignore or discount them, things may improve. Similarly, the Fire child might recognize that the stodginess of Earth parents is in need of motivation and inspiration from the offspring. If the child turns his or her energy to inspiring them and including them in his or her world of experience, rather than in rebellion, the relationship will be eased.

Whatever your situation, it can be countered or improved with a few simple recommendations. Always carry a vial of your favorite elemental scent. Use it as an inhalant when you feel your energies begin to wane or when hostilities rise. Wear something of your element color to work everyday, and instead of gulping down those gallons of coffee or soda, try brewing a tea made of your elemental herbs.

Have an unpredictable lover? Why not purchase a beautiful robe or sheets in a color scheme compatible with both your ruling energies? Parents or kids driving you nuts? Paint your bedroom in a color compatible with your personal energy field. Go there to nourish yourself and meditate when you can. If you can't, try the old rose-colored glasses trick: Simple sunglasses are tinted in a variety of shades these days, and you can certainly find a pair tinted in your elemental color. Wear them to "change your perspective."

Finally, always carry a personal power stone or piece of jewelry that has been annointed with essential oil somewhere on your person. For particularly stressful periods, combine that stone with a piece of clear or rose quartz.

Astrological Keys

FOR A MORE COMPREHENSIVE VIEW OF YOUR OWN OR
someone else's elemental ruler, first consider the sign,
elemental ruler, and house placement of the sun,
moon, and rising signs. Obviously, someone born under
the sign of Leo, with the moon in Aries and Sagittarius
rising, is ruled predominantly by the element of Fire. A
Libra with Pisces rising and a Cancer moon, on the
other hand, is under a Water rulership, while retaining
some Airier qualities. But should that same Libra have
Venus and Mercury in Scorpio and a Pluto/Moon
conjunction, the Air influence can be pinpointed as
entirely subordinate to the heavier Water influence and
perhaps in need of regular healing and augmentation,
so that the more intellectual aspects of this personality
are not consistently overwhelmed by its more emotional
qualities.

In determining the elemental rulers of the individual chart, several secondary factors—beyond the

primary placement of the sun, moon, and rising signs—must be taken into account. These include determining those elements governing the sign and house placement of any stellium—or planetary cluster—apparent in the chart, and considering also whether or not a horoscope shows a critical placement of one or more of the outer planets—a Saturn/Neptune conjunction on the mid-heaven, for example. The elements governing Sun, Moon, Mars, Mercury, Jupiter, and Venus can be said to speak to an individual's attunement to elemental energy on a conscious level. The elements governing Saturn, Neptune, and Pluto will give the interpreter an idea of the way in which that individual is subconsciously attuned to the Universal Energy. Someone with the inner planets placed primarily in Fire and outer planets in Water is going to deal with the world in a Fiery fashion—enthusiastic, passionate, and impatient. Their subconscious attunement, however, is going to lead them to a certain amount of acting out a deep-seated, subconscious need for emotional security.

Look also at squares and oppositions in the chart. A Sun/Mars conjunction in an Air sign opposite a Fire-ruled rising sign will in effect "fuel" that personality's Fiery approach to the world—Air feeds Fire. On the other hand, a Pluto/Moon conjunction in Water square a Fiery sun will do much to dampen and repress the natural energy and enthusiasm of Fire.

Finally, it will be especially useful to look at the planetary placement in the houses as defined by their elemental rulership.

The Elemental House Rulerships

Water: The Fourth, Eighth, and Twelfth Houses

Each of these houses concern themselves with "Watery" issues of security and insecurity, and with the individual's ability or inability to assimilate emotional experience. The fourth rules the parental home and the need for privacy. The eighth is security through material values and the need to experience emotional contact—the ultimate intimacy as expressed in sex and psychic knowledge. The twelfth house is growth through insecurity—gradual awareness gained through events beyond our control and the assimilation of past-life experience.

Earth: The Second, Sixth, and Tenth Houses

The Earth houses rule the issues tied to the material world, and speak to an individual's ability to cope with material affairs in a physical universe. The second house rules money, acquisitions, and a sense of material security. The sixth rules learning by experience in the material world and its limitations. The tenth rules self-directed action in the material world, vocation, and reputation.

Fire: The First, Fifth, and Ninth Houses

Fire houses can be said to represent the range of self-discovery as presented by the Fire issues of personal identity, creativity, and knowledge. The first house rules appearance on one level, but also can be said to rule, at a deeper level, the individual's sense of self. The fifth house rules creativity, romance, and children but is also expressive of the individual's ability to share their identity with others through those forms of expression. The ninth house governs knowledge, philosophy, and religion—that is, the ability to identify one's place and meaning in a larger context, i.e., "I know who I am—why am I here?"

Air: The Third, Seventh, and Eleventh Houses

Air houses are concerned with the area and range of relationship as governed by the Air issues of communication, social urges, and intellectual needs. The third house rules basic communications skills, but is also representative of early socialization in the form of siblings. The seventh rules partnership issues, marriage, and one-on-one communications. The eleventh house rules the search for social acceptance and security, group alignment, and shared ideas.

Thus, the placement of planets in the houses will significantly affect the elemental operatives in a chart. A Watery Sun/Moon conjunction in Pisces, for example, will be significantly altered by its placement in the third house. Such a person's Watery inuitive energy will be better expressed and more easily communicated than is usual for Water-ruled personalities—probably due to their having been born into a large family or through some other significant form of early socialization. A concentration of Fire in the twelfth house will bespeak an individual somewhat short on self-awareness but whose life and needs are intimately tied to events beyond their control. A Watery moon in the fifth house will show a romantic emotional approach to love; an Airy Mercury in the second will show someone who makes money from his verbal gifts.

Any good astrological computer chart will offer you an elemental breakdown of the planets in their signs and houses, but your own intuition should also have a role in determining the core personality of yourself and others. Keep in mind that these elements came to be associated with personality and destiny because they were seen, over and over again, to correspond with certain qualities of soul.

Interpreting Your Elements

You will need a good computer program or chart to delineate your natal data. I especially recommend ASTRO for Windows by Christopher J. Noyes, copyright 1993, though there are a number of fine astrology programs out there. If you prefer, use the services of a good professional astrologer.

To make it easier for the individual to understand where and how the elements fit together in a chart, let's assign a simple point system to the elements of the individual horoscope.

Sun = 20 points
Moon = 10 points
Rising Sign = 10 points
Mercury = 5 points
Venus = 5 points
Mars = 5 points
Jupiter = 10 points
Saturn = 10 points
Uranus = 10 points
Neptune = 10 points
Pluto = 10 points

Stellium (three or more planets in one sign or house): add 10 points
Conjunctions: add 5 points
Midheaven and Immum Coeli: 5 points each
Trines to similar elements: add 5 points
Squares: subtract 10

Start by adding up the point value of your planets in the elements. For example, let's look at the elemental value of a sample chart, that of President Bill Clinton.

Bill Clinton:
8/19/1946
7:30 A.M.
Little Rock, AK
33.40 N 93.35 W

RISING SIGN: Virgo (10 points Earth)
SUN: Leo (20 points Fire)
MOON: Taurus (10 points Earth)
MERCURY: Leo (5 points Fire)
VENUS: Libra (5 points Air)
MARS: Libra (5 points Air)
JUPITER: Libra (10 points Air)
SATURN: Leo (10 points Fire)
URANUS: Gemini (10 points Air)
NEPTUNE: Libra (10 points Air)
PLUTO: Leo (10 points Fire)

Thus at first glance, Mr. Clinton's elemental profile works up like this:

EARTH: 20 points
FIRE: 55 points
AIR: 45 points
WATER: 0 points

Yet a closer look at Mr. Clinton's chart will yield two important facts. First, his Earthy Virgo rising is in fact squared to his Uranus in Gemini in the midheaven, lessening the importance of the Earth energy in his chart. And, second, his Mercury is conjunct to two of the most important outer planets—Saturn and Pluto in the Fire sign of Leo—making for a stellium in the eleventh house, quite near his sun, yet not actually conjunct to it. With Uranus on his midheaven in Airy Gemini, squared to earth rising, it exerts considerable influence on how Mr. Clinton would like the world to perceive him and his work. So, adding the value of those configurations, the point value of the elements comes out like this:

EARTH: 20 points
FIRE: 75 points
AIR: 50 points
WATER: 0 points

Clearly Mr. Clinton can be defined as a Fire-ruled personality, with a prominent, though not necessarily dominant, Air influence.

Let's consider another personality type:

11/13/56
11:30 A.M.
Binghamton, NY
42.06 N 75.54 W

RISING SIGN: Capricorn (10 points Earth)
SUN: Scorpio (20 points Water)
MOON: Pisces (10 points Water)
MERCURY: Scorpio (5 points Water)
VENUS: Libra (5 points Air)
MARS: Pisces (5 points Water)
JUPITER: Virgo (10 points Earth)

SATURN: Sagittarius (10 points Fire)
URANUS: Leo (10 points Fire)
NEPTUNE: Cusp between Libra and Scorpio
(5 points each Air and Water)
PLUTO: On the cusp between Virgo and Leo
(5 points each for Earth and Fire)

The elemental breakdown of the chart is as follows:

EARTH: 25 points
FIRE: 25 points
AIR: 10 points
WATER: 45 points

It would be perhaps too obvious to call this person a Water-ruled personality—there are simply too many elemental influences going on for Water to be called really dominant in the chart. To get a clearer idea of what the true ruling influence is in this person's life, then, let's take another look at the chart.

The sun in this particular chart is in the tenth house, almost conjunct with the midheaven in Scorpio; add another ten points for Water. Further, the elemental influence of the two powerful outer planets Neptune and Pluto is considerably weakened by their cusp placement. While many astrologers would argue that the transitional placement of these two planets is critical to interpreting the chart as a whole, keep in mind that we are talking about kinds of energy here—not predictive or interpretive astrology per se.

That is why our point system assigns a lesser value to the inner planets. Their frequent transits certainly affect our day-to-day activities but not as much our essential nature or energy patterns. The outer planets, on the other hand, have a great elemental value in determining our element. That is why astrologers concern themselves so greatly with the transits of these planets. If Pluto moves, as it has quite recently done, from Scorpio to Sagittarius, world events and whole patterns of energy change. Our friend the Scorpio above is going to feel rather "out of her element" as a result.

Does a secondary study of the chart above still reveal a Water-ruled personality? Yes. But she is perhaps a more motivated and practical Water-type than some others. A final word about this sample chart: The planet Venus—which rules attraction, love, and beauty, among other things—is without aspects to the rest of the horoscope. It is also in the element of Air. From a purely elemental point of view, then, it should be said that her Watery emotional nature is not going to be much influenced by trying to "balance" her energy with Air. Instead, this individual will literally find healing by associating and establishing relationships with those who have a prominent Air energy. What is a woman like this going to look for in a man? Intelligence, ideals, and the ability to verbalize them well.

Still, in both of the examples above, it's worth noting that the ruling element of the sun sign does in fact turn out to be the ruling element of the personality. But if you or someone else feels that their true nature is not at all described by their elemental profile, you may want to make a deeper interpretive analysis.

Crystal and Aromatherapy Keys

Gems and Minerals Associated to the Elements

USE THE LIST BELOW AS A GUIDE TO SELECTING THE STONES and minerals most compatible with your elemental ruler. Always be aware that intuition and personal attraction should be your primary reasons for choosing a particular stone for healing purposes though, and that we are attracted to different stones and their energies at different times. When a stone has outlived its usefulness for you, put it away, or, better still, pass it on to a trusted friend or loved one.

EARTH STONES AND MINERALS

Tiger's eye
Jet
Black or white onyx
Amethyst
Lapis lazuli
Petrified wood
Sapphire and star sapphire
Citrine
Emerald
Amber
Royal azel
Limestone
Loadstone
Moss agate

WATER STONES AND MINERALS

Aventurine
Tourmaline or beryl
Marble
Coral
Pearl
Abalone
Turquoise
Topaz
Moonstone
Picture agate
Malachite
Obsidian
Opal
Garnet
Rhodonite

FIRE STONES AND MINERALS

Soapstone
Ivory
Fire agate
Diamond
Bloodstone
Creedite
Azurite
Pink tourmaline
Amber
Ruby
Red onyx
Carnelian
Pyrite or fool's gold
Sardonyx
Sandstone

AIR STONES AND MINERALS

Alexandrite
Apatite
Peridot
Chrysocolla
Chrysopase
Chrysolite
Rholodite
Blue sapphire
Lazulite
Jade
Herkimer diamond
Serpentine
Titanite
Flint
Fluorite

Birthstones

The following is a list of traditional birthstones according to month:

January—Garnet
February—Amethyst
March—Bloodstone
April—Diamond
May—Emerald
June—Pearl
July—Turquoise
August—Sardonyx
September—Peridot
October—Beryl
November—Topaz
December—Ruby

Metals and Energy Corresponding to the Signs of the Zodiac

ARIES: Iron, carbon steel
TAURUS: Copper
GEMINI: Molybdenum
CANCER: Silver
LEO: Gold
VIRGO: Magnesium
LIBRA: Palladium
SCORPIO: Manganese
SAGITTARIUS: Tin
CAPRICORN: Zinc
AQUARIUS: Chromium
PISCES: Platinum

The Houses of the Zodiac and Their Associated Gemstones

Note your chart and see where the concentration of planets are placed in the twelve houses. Using this list you may augment your personal power stones with the appropriate house stones in healing or use them to concentrate on a particular area of your life that you feel requires extra healing energy. Need money? Carry a lapis lazuli. Upset over some old family issues? Keep a moonstone at hand. . . . Whatever the problem or area of concern, refer to this list often for special healing.

FIRST HOUSE: Coral
SECOND HOUSE: Lapis lazuli
THIRD HOUSE: Picture agate
FOURTH HOUSE: Moonstone
FIFTH HOUSE: Yellow jasper
SIXTH HOUSE: Star sapphire
SEVENTH HOUSE: Emerald
EIGHTH HOUSE: Dark opal
NINTH HOUSE: Turquoise
TENTH HOUSE: Clear quartz
ELEVENTH HOUSE: Garnet
TWELFTH HOUSE: Light opal

Stones for Any Sign or Element

These stones are generally favored for their all-purpose usefulness, purifying energies, and calming effects. Quartz particularly is thought to enhance the power of other stones when carried or worn in conjunction with them.

Quartz
Rose quartz
Smoky quartz
Coral
Loadstone
Diamond
Turquoise

Crystals and Aromatherapy

Many practitioners believe that the powers of a particular gemstone or crystal are enhanced by the application of one of more drops of essential oil. On the following page is a brief reference list of compatible oils and stones for each of the four elements. They constitute only a few of the possibilities for combining the powers of your stones and scent for healing purposes. Remember that only essential oils—that is, commercially distilled and highly concentrated essences—are to be used for these purposes. Ensure their effectiveness by dealing with a reputable dealer or aromatherapist. See Appendix on page 217. Experiment with these combinations or combine your choice of oils and stones for specific effects and energies.

To consecrate the stone of your choice for healing purposes, choose a day when the sun and moon are both in a sign of your personal element. For example, a Fire-ruled personality could choose a day when the sun is in Sagittarius and the moon is in the sign of Leo or Aries. A basic method for anointing stones to increase their powers is as follows:

> Hold the stone and feel its energy field aligning with your own. It may help you to visualize the energy coursing up through your hand to your arm, up to your shoulder, and radiating through the rest of your body. Inhale the fragrance of the essential oil of your choice deeply; imagine its scent vibrating in accord with the energy of your crystal or stone.

Hold the energy within your being; feel its warmth and power. Anoint the stone by placing a drop of the essential oil on the stone (preferably on the matrix) and carry the stone with you for as long as you deem necessary.

GEMSTONE OR CRYSTAL	ESSENCE	HEALING FUNCTION
Amethyst	Yarrow	psychic power
Carnelian	Cardamom	sexual problems
Aquamarine	Eucalyptus	purification
Rhodochrosite	Ginger	physical energy
Moonstone	Jasmine	insomnia, love
Fluorite	Lavender	health, consciousness
Malachite	Pine	money, protection
Rose Quartz	Rose	happiness, joy
Tourmaline	Patchouli	money, protection
Calcite	Sandalwood	spirituality
Kunzite	Ylang-ylang	inner peace
Quartz crystal	Rosemary	positive change

Elemental Herb and Essence Association Keys

EARTH

Balm of Gilead
Bistort
Black pepper
Cedar
Cinquefoil
Cypress
Fern
High John the
    Conqueror
Honeysuckle
Horehound
Jasmine
Mandrake
Mimosa
Myrrh
Patchouli
Pine
Sage
Slippery elm
Thyme
Tonka beans

WATER

Apple
Ash
Burdock
Camphor
Chamomile
Catnip
Cyclamen
Gardenia
Hawthorn
Heather
Hyacinth
Hyssop
Jasmine
Henbane
Hops
Ivy
Lovage
Lily
Meadowsweet
Mock or sweet orange
Myrtle
Orris
Pansy
Periwinkle
Pennyroyal
Palmarosa
Poppy
Rose
Sandalwood
Violet
Thyme
Willow
Ylang-ylang

FIRE

Angelica
Bergamot
Basil
Bay
Calendula
Clove
Carnation
Celandine
Coriander
Cumin
Frankincense
Garlic
Ginger
Heliotrope
Holly
Juniper
Lemon
Lime
Marigold
Nasturtium
Neroli
Nutmeg
Peony
Pennyroyal
Saffron
St. John's wort

AIR

Acacia
Anise
Benzoin
Caraway
Comfrey
Daffodil
Dill
Elder
Eucalyptus
Fennel
Geranium
Hazel
Lavender
Lemongrass
Lemon verbena
Lily of the valley
Marjoram
Mint
Mistletoe
Parsley
Rosemary
Peppermint
Sweet pea

Appendices

Appendices

Sources of Supplies and Information

The American Aromatherapy Association
P.O. Box 1222
Fair Oaks, CA 95628

Aromatherapy International
P.O. Box 3679
South Pasadena, CA 91031

Aphrodisia
282 Bleecker Street
New York, NY 10018
(dried plants and herbs)

Aroma Vera
P.O. Box 3609
Culver City, CA 90231
(213) 280-0407

Companion Plants
724 North Coolville Ridge Road
Athens, OH 45701

Enchantments
341 East 9th Street
New York, NY 10013

Herbal Endeavors
3618 South Emmons Avenue
Rochester Hills, MI
(313) 852-0796

Original Swiss Aromatics
P.O. Box 606
San Rafael, CA 94915

Bibliography and Suggested Reading

Arroyo, Stephen. *Astrology, Psychology and the Four Elements*, CRCS Publications, Sebastopol, CA, 1975.

Crawford, E. A., and Kennedy, Teresa. *Chinese Elemental Astrology*, NAL Books, New York, 1990.

Cunningham, Scott. *Magical Aromatherapy*, Lllewellyn, St. Paul, MN, 1994.

Cunningham, Scott. *Magical Herbalism*, Lllewellyn, St. Paul, MN, 1985.

Hunt, Roland. *The Seven Keys to Color Healing*, Harper and Row, New York, 1982.

Huson, Paul. *Mastering Herbalism*, Stein and Day, Briarcliff Manor, NY, 1983.

Lust, John. *The Herb Book*, Bantam Books, New York, 1974.

McCarthy, Paul. *A Beginner's Guide to Shiatsu*, Avery Publishing Group, Garden City Park, New York, 1995.

The Prevention How-to Dictionary of Healing Remedies and Techniques, MJF Books, New York, 1992.

Ryman, Daniele. *Aromatherapy*, Bantam Books, New York, 1991.

Sullivan, Kevin. *The Crystal Handbook*, NAL Books, New York, 1987.